Palo Alto City Library

The individual borrower is responsible for all library material borrowed on his or her card.

Charges as determined by the CITY OF PALO ALTO will be assessed for each overdue item.

Damaged or non-returned property will be billed to the individual borrower by the CITY OF PALO ALTO.

P.O. Box 10250, Palo Alto, CA 94303

Natural
Highs

Other books by Dr. Hyla Cass

Kava: Nature's Answer to Stress, Anxiety, and Insomnia (with Terrence McNally)

St. John's Wort: Nature's Blues Buster

User's Guide to Ginkgo

User's Guide to Vitamin C (with Jim English)

Other books by Patrick Holford

The Optimum Nutrition Bible

100% Health

The Optimum Nutrition Cookbook (with Judy Ridgway)

6 Weeks to Superhealth

Balancing Hormones Naturally (with Kate Neil)

Beat Stress and Fatigue

Boost Your Immune System (with Jennifer Meek)

Improve Your Digestion

Say No to Cancer

Say No to Heart Disease

Say No to Arthritis

The 30 Day Fat Burner Diet

Supplements for Superhealth

The Little Book of Optimum Nutrition

Solve Your Skin Problems (with Natalie Savona)

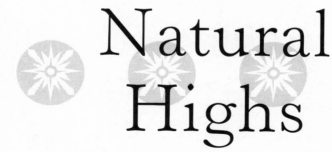

Natural Highs

SUPPLEMENTS, NUTRITION,

AND MIND-BODY TECHNIQUES

TO HELP YOU FEEL GOOD

ALL THE TIME

Hyla Cass, M.D.
and Patrick Holford

Avery

a member of

Penguin Putnam Inc.

New York

a member of
Penguin Putnam Inc.
375 Hudson Street
New York, NY 10014
www.penguinputnam.com

Library of Congress Cataloging-in-Publication Data
Cass, Hyla.
Natural highs : supplements, nutrition, and mind-body techniques to help you
feel good all the time / [Hyla Cass and Patrick Holford].
p.   cm.
Includes bibliographical references and index.
ISBN 1-58333-133-6
1. Naturopathy.   2. Mind and body.   3. Dietary supplements.
4. Nutrition.   I. Holford, Patrick.   II. Title.
[DNLM: 1. Stress, Psychological—therapy.   2. Complementary Therapies.
3. Mind-Body and Relaxation Techniques—methods.   4. Naturopathy.   5. Nutrition.
WM 172 C343n 2002]
RZ440 .C344   2002   2001056705
615.5'35—dc21

Printed in the United States of America
1   3   5   7   9   10   8   6   4   2

This book is printed on acid-free paper. ♾

Book design by Meighan Cavanaugh

Illustrations by Jim English and Jonathan Phillips

Acknowledgments

This book would not have been possible without the help and support of many people. We would both like to thank Ken Blum, Ph.D., Jerry Cott, Ph.D., Charles Grob, M.D., Abram Hoffer, M.D., Ann Shulgin, Alexander (Sasha) Shulgin, Ph.D., and Rick Strassman, M.D., for their guidance and research input.

I would like to thank Jeremy Tarcher, who first sparked to the idea; Joel Fotinos at Tarcher, who adopted it; John Duff at Avery and the editorial team, who saw it through to completion. Special thanks to Executive Editor Laura Shepherd, who shared my vision, was endlessly supportive, and did an incredible job of editing. Thanks, too, to copyeditor Carol Rosenberg. Thanks to my family, including my mother, Miriam; my three sisters and their husbands; and my daughter, Alison, and my son-in-law, Seth. Thanks also to my many friends who advised and supported me.

Special thanks to Terrence McNally, who helped me to write and rewrite, was always available for feedback, and reminded me to take a break now and then; and to Jim English, who, besides doing a great job on the diagrams, had the gift of understanding my meaning and helped me to communicate it more artfully. Above all, I thank my patients, who have trusted me with their well-being and have taught me what I know.

—*Hyla Cass*

I would like to thank Oscar Ichazo and many other people who have helped with guidance and research; and Bebe Kohlap for taking care of things during my absences. Very special thanks go to Natalie Savona for help with editing and to Rachel Winning and her team at Piatkus, especially Barbara Kiser, for their painstaking editing and design.

—*Patrick Holford*

Contents

PART THREE: LIVING HIGH NATURALLY

PART FOUR: NATURAL HIGHS AT A GLANCE

Introduction

Imagine living in a world where you feel happy, alert, and energetic more often than not—a place where feeling "high" and at one with the world is the norm, where getting high is healthy and nonaddictive. Does this sound like science fiction? As we'll see, it can be as simple as child's play, where it all begins.

Pass any playground full of five- or six-year-olds, and you are immediately struck by the bubbling energy that radiates from this running, laughing, shouting sea of children. They embrace the world and interact with it in a way that many of us have forgotten. We seldom find a young child who is the least bit shy about singing, dancing, or drawing in front of others. But how many of us would even contemplate doing the same?

Spontaneous and positive, children are naturally high. They will go out of their way to enhance this, too, by swinging on swings or spinning in circles until they collapse. Even their crying and angry outbursts are an essential part of this spontaneity. As we approach adolescence, however, we become "socialized" and lose some of this seemingly innate capacity for fun and pleasure.

As adults, we adopt repetitive and rote behaviors; we surrender and become numb to life. We forget to smell the flowers (sensory awareness), appreciate our loved ones (an open heart), and take pleasure in finding new ways of doing things (mental flexibility). But are these losses inevitable? Is it possible for us to experience the open, spontaneous, and energetic joy we once had? In *Natural Highs,* we discuss how we can once again embrace this more childlike state. One vital key to sustaining mood, energy, and connection is to be aware, present, and open to new ideas, behaviors, and perceptions.

In the following chapters, you'll discover everything you need to experience a natural, childlike high. We include a range of techniques and nutrients designed to promote sensory awareness and mental flexibility, as well as to restore and maintain your energy level. You'll then be able to find your own perfect combination of diet, nutrients, and activities for staying naturally high, including:

- Hangover-free alternatives to relaxing with a beer, martini, or a glass of wine.
- Natural, nonaddictive ways to get the same energy kick that you get from coffee, tea, or tobacco.
- Safe, natural, and effective alternatives to Prozac and Valium, with no side effects.
- Natural nutrients to help take you to higher states of awareness and connection, without the side effects of drugs.
- Nourishing foods that can replenish and restore your brain, depleted by stress or excessive drug and alcohol use.
- Natural substances that help you escape addictions, including some that you may not even realize you have.

You'll quickly see that getting high can be healthy, nonaddictive, and as easy as taking a quick trip to the supermarket, drugstore, or health food store.

Altering Mind, Mood, and Energy

At this point you may be questioning whether it is even *natural* to feel this good all the time! It certainly isn't the norm in our culture. And, in fact, evidence suggests that depression and anxiety may offer evolutionary advantages. Our ancestors knew that maintaining an edge and keeping a vigilant eye out for enemies had great survival value. Being too blissed-out might make you some predator's dinner! Despite the absence of this ongoing threat, many of us are still on edge, anxious, and/or depressed. If this sounds like you, the good news is that there are natural, mind-altering supplements and techniques that can help you to break your patterns and create new and happier responses to life's inevitable changes, disappointments, and surprises.

Of course, "natural" can mean a lot of things these days. Coffee, alcohol, nicotine, marijuana, and even cocaine all are provided by Mother Nature, but they're not on our recommended list. By natural, we mean substances that are both legal and good for you. Such substances work with your body's design, not against it. Used correctly, they can balance and increase health and energy rather than deplete it.

Feel-good substances permeate our culture. In an average week, Americans drink 3.4 million cups of tea, 1 billion cups of coffee, 4.5 billion sugared and/or caffeinated soft drinks, 2.3 billion alcoholic drinks; smoke 8.25 billion cigarettes; and consume 845,726,369 pounds (or about 420,000 tons) of sugar and 20 million pounds of chocolate. On top of this we take 20 million antidepressants, puff our way through 25 million joints, and pop 1 million tabs of Ecstasy.

All that popping, pouring, and puffing wouldn't be so popular unless it worked. In fact, these substances can boost our energy, relieve our anxiety, help us recover from a hard day's work, and escape our less than perfect reality. Unfortunately, these highs evaporate all too quickly, leaving us to cope with a nasty aftermath of mood swings, emotional depletion, physical exhaustion, and even addiction. If you've quit, that's probably why. And if you haven't, it's probably why you're reading this book.

Take Me Higher: Spirit and Transcendence

"High" has many meanings and connotations, which range from the just-mentioned chemical variety to the way we feel when we fall in love, see a magnificent sunset, or ride a roller coaster; to the energy and exuberance most of us had as children; or to another dimension entirely—the realm of transcendent or "peak" experiences. We feel high when we experience a profound sense of unity and harmony, a deep connection with others, and a shared sense of life's purpose. This is the flash of inspiration, the epiphany that fuels great works of music, art, and poetry, as well as scientific and spiritual breakthroughs.

What's more, this shared human experience of connection with nature, the universe, or God, while often difficult to describe in words, can actually be measured by a brain scan. Researchers have isolated a small portion of the emotional center of the brain that is the most active when we are having a spiritual experience. We may actually be hardwired for this essential connection, with that area being a special receiving or connecting point. Scientists can even induce such experiences by electrically stimulating that portion of the brain, which Dr. Michael Persinger at Laurentian University refers to as "the God module."

Some fear that such research, which gives spiritual experience an anatomical location, reduces its deeper significance. Others are excited by the concept, which seems to prove the reality of this near-universal experience. Whatever your interpretation, though, it implies that if you have a functioning brain, you are very likely able to experience a spiritual high.

Traditional cultures all over the world have used psychoactive drugs to attain these peak states. We substitute various herbal combinations that you can use to alter your mind-state. They also used specific methods, such as meditation, movement, drumming, visualization, or special breathing techniques that you will find in Part Three.

How We Work: The Mind-Body Connection

These mood-enhancing techniques depend on the mind-body connection, with brain chemistry as the link. One of the most exciting new areas of medical science, the study of the "mind-body" interface, is helping us to understand for the first time just how this works, and what you and I can do to improve our minds and moods.

This topic has fascinated both of us for more than twenty years. In our professional experience as a psychiatrist and as a nutritionist specializing in mental health problems, we have worked with hundreds of clients with serious emotional problems. By helping them modify their brain chemistry, we have witnessed remarkable recoveries to robust mental health. We've found that certain natural substances can pull you out of depression, restore balance in times of stress, or promote an exhilarating sense of well-being.

We have also come across many people, especially those approaching middle age (it happens to the best of us), who have an additional problem. They are less able to tolerate the use of alcohol, marijuana, or other relaxants or stimulants that they once used freely. Others complain that the effect is diminished, that it "just isn't what it used to be." To their dismay, many have also noticed that their long-term substance use, even if it was only intermittent, has affected their mental abilities.

> *Noel, a forty-five-year-old stockbroker and long-time pot smoker, complained, "Not only doesn't it work as well as it once did, but I feel so tired and foggy the next day that the temporary high is just not worth it. My memory isn't as good as it used to be, either."*
>
> *Fortunately, with the regular use of some prescribed supplements, Noel regained his mental faculties and energy. In fact, he claimed, "I haven't felt this clear and energetic since I was in my twenties!" In the process, he also lost his desire for smoking pot.*

When you substitute "pot" with alcohol, cigarettes, coffee, or any other mind- and mood-altering substance, then you have an idea of the scope of the problem and the effectiveness of our solution. This sounds miraculous, and it is. As researchers unravel how natural mind-altering substances change our perceptions and moods, they've discovered an amazing thing: almost all of these substances are similar to our own brain chemicals and seem to work by mimicking, boosting, or blocking their effects.

What this means, of course, is that we are all theoretically capable of producing our own natural highs, without even taking the substance. How? The answer lies deep in our brains, with those chemical messengers of mind and emotions, the *neurotransmitters* (discussed in detail in Chapter 2).

Since neurotransmitters are literally made from nutrients—amino acids, vitamins, and minerals—we can formulate the perfect "brain food" to improve how we feel and think. Nutritional supplements can create a state of high energy, increased focus, and good mood. With the right combinations, well-being, connection, and *joie de vivre* can become your normal state of mind.

Feeding your brain is vital. Just as important is remembering that chemistry works both ways: various substances can promote a natural high, *and* positive states of mind can raise your "happy" brain chemicals. Our mind power is a remarkable, often untapped resource in our search for happiness.

How to Use This Book

Part One consists of three chapters, starting with the Natural High Questionnaires. These questionnaires will help you assess your own current needs, habits, and patterns and to develop your own strategy for shifting to natural highs.

We then introduce you to the basics of brain function. You will learn about neurotransmitters, the brain's "communication chemicals" that are capable of stimulating and relaxing you, lifting your mood, and sharpening your mind. You will find out why some substances knock your chemistry out of balance, while others are good for you. We then give you the Natural High Basics, a core regimen of food and supplements that creates the best internal environment for sustaining mood and energy. You will learn how to support your brain and body chemistry for maximum energy and balance.

Part Two is the heart of the book—six chapters that deal with the issues and substances that probably attracted you to this book in the first place: Stress Busters, Energizers, Mood Enhancers, Mind and Memory Boosters, Making the Connection, and Addiction.

Each chapter presents its information in the following sequence:

- How you would prefer to feel, and how you might be feeling now.
- What goes on in your body and brain chemistry when you feel this way.
- The upsides and downsides of conventional substances that we use, such as alcohol and tranquilizers.

Introduction

- The natural alternatives that can produce the desired result without the downsides. We'll learn why they work, the research on their benefits, and how to use them.
- Finally, there's a straightforward action plan—clear and simple steps to achieve a natural high.

Part Three suggests other ways to achieve your natural high. You will see how breathing, meditation, exercise, and sleep can raise mood and energy. We also look at positive thinking, sex, and the life-enhancing uses of music, light, color, and aromatherapy.

Part Four offers top tips on natural ways to chill out, boost your energy, lift your mood, enhance your mind, and get connected. There is also an A to Z listing of the substances you can take to achieve a natural high.

GUIDE TO ABBREVIATIONS AND MEASURES

1 gram (g) = 1,000 milligrams (mg) = 1,000,000 micrograms (mcg)

Part One

GETTING IN
THE MOOD

How Naturally High Are You?

We believe it is possible to be high—firing on all cylinders, inspired, enthusiastic, happy, calm, and alert—much of the time. Our Natural High Program shows you how to sustain the right biochemical, physical, and psychological conditions. There are four steps to being naturally high:

1. *Achieve optimum brain nutrition.*

A good diet and the right supplements provide you with the necessary building blocks for brain cells and neurotransmitters, which are the mood, mind, and memory molecules. You will also be able to balance your blood sugar, which acts as brain and body fuel. This helps you to break your dependency on substances that interfere with normal brain chemistry and deplete your energy.

2. *Keep yourself "fine-tuned" with natural highs.*

The reality of day-to-day life is that you will likely become stressed out or otherwise unbalanced. You will learn how to use natural substances to help bring yourself back into balance.

3. *Think positively.*

Chemistry isn't the whole story when it comes to natural highs. It's also about how we think. Ironically, while fear and anxiety seem to come easily, we often have to work harder to achieve happiness. Fortunately, you can replace negative patterns with a more positive and uplifting frame of mind.

4. *Adopt a naturally high lifestyle.*

There are many ways to improve how you feel, specific lifestyle changes in the form of physical, mental, emotional, and spiritual exercises.

The Natural High Program is designed to help you make and maintain the step-by-step changes in your life that will allow you to be naturally and consistently high.

Before leaping headfirst into the mass of information that follows, check out the following Natural High Questionnaires, which will help you to develop your personal natural high strategy.

The Natural High Questionnaires

Each of us is unique—an amalgam of genetic inheritance and a lifetime of experience. We may have inherited certain tendencies, for example, toward depression or anxiety. These tendencies, together with what we have learned in childhood, and indulged in as adults, have programmed our body chemistry. This is turn affects our behavior. We may find ourselves, for instance, with a nonstop need for stimulation or a seemingly built-in inability to relax.

The good news is that none of this is set in stone. You *can* change.

The Natural High Questionnaires will help you to figure out what you need to work on. In each of the following questionnaires, mark "yes" if the question applies more than half of the time. Score one point for each "yes" answer.

HOW STRESSED ARE YOU?

This questionnaire will help you recognize some of the signs and see where you fit on the stress continuum.

- Do you have difficulty relaxing? ____
- Do you often feel irritable? ____
- Do you worry about the little events of the day, and find that you are unable to shut off your mind? ____
- Do you smoke or drink excessively (especially by other people's standards)? ____
- Are you competitive and aggressive? ____
- Do you find it hard to relate to people? ____
- Do you find yourself impatient with others? ____
- Do you eat quickly? ____
- Do you take on too much? ____
- Do you have difficulty delegating? ____
- Do you have aching limbs, tense muscles, or recurrent headaches? ____
- Do you have a dry mouth and sweaty palms? ____
- Do you feel a lack of interest in sex? ____
- Do you have problems sleeping? ____

Scoring

1–5: Like most of us, you could use some practical ideas on how to calm down when challenges arise. Or you may want to reach states of even deeper peace. If so, read on for some inspiring ideas.

6–10: You are quite stressed. Pay attention to these warning signs. This is the only body you have. Treat it well. You'll see how to do this in the following pages.

11–14: You are very stressed. Clean up your act before there are serious consequences. Turn to Chapter 4 to find out how.

ENERGY CHECK

To get an idea of how depleted your energy might be and how dependent you are on stimulants, check yourself out in the following questionnaire.

- Do you have trouble getting up in the morning? ___
- Do you rely on a cup of coffee to get you going in the morning? ___
- Do you feel tired all the time? ___
- Do you often feel foggy, fuzzy, or dull? ___
- Do you have trouble concentrating? ___
- Do you use sugar, caffeine (tea, coffee, caffeinated soft drinks), or a cigarette as a pick-me-up throughout the day? ___
- Are you often irritable or angry for no apparent reason? ___
- Do your moods seem to go up and down for no apparent reason? ___
- Are your mood swings often relieved by food, especially sweets? ___
- Do you have trouble falling asleep at night? ___
- Do you have headaches or shaky feelings that are relieved by sugar, caffeine, or cigarettes? ___
- Do you suspect you're addicted to coffee, caffeinated soft drinks, or cigarettes? ___
- Do you find yourself constantly in crisis? ___
- Are you drawn to thrills, danger, and drama in your life? ___

Scoring
   1–5: We all have our moments—bad moods, feeling tired or foggy, and in need of a pick-me-up, but there may be some warning signs for you here.
   6–10: You are showing signs of depleted energy and may even be overly dependent on stimulants to keep you going. Chapter 5 will explain what is happening in your body and how to make healthier choices.
   11–14: You are quite depleted and at risk for becoming hooked on stimulants. It is affecting your mental and physical health. You can get off them with the right diet, supplement, and lifestyle changes. We will show you how in Chapter 9.

MOOD CHECK

See where you fit on the continuum from happy and content to blue, all the way down to clinically depressed. (No one but you will be looking at the answers, so be honest!)

- Do you feel downhearted, blue, and sad? ____
- Do you feel worse in the morning? ____
- Do you have crying spells or often feel like crying? ____
- Do you have trouble falling asleep or sleeping through the night? ____
- Is your appetite poor, or are you losing weight without trying? ____
- Are you overeating and/or gaining weight? ____
- Do you feel unattractive and unlovable? ____
- Do you prefer to be alone? ____
- Do you feel fearful? ____
- Are you often tired and irritable? ____
- Is it an effort to do the things you used to do with ease? ____
- Do you feel hopeless about the future? ____
- Do you find it difficult to make decisions? ____
- Do you feel less enjoyment from activities that once gave you pleasure? ____

Scoring:

1–5: You are normal, usually able to roll with the punches. Chapter 6 will give you clues on how to handle those occasions when things *aren't* going so well for you.

6–10: You have a mild to moderate case of the blues. Read on to see how this can happen, and then, to the solutions.

11–14: You are moderately to markedly depressed. Besides reading Chapter 6, consider seeking professional help.

If you were in the depressed range, you should start by consulting your physician or health practitioner to make sure there is no physical cause for your problems. Then, unless you are fortunate to have someone who does both, consult a psychotherapist and a natural medicine practitioner (see the

Resources section). A psychotherapist will deal with psychological issues, while a natural medicine practitioner will help to find any underlying chemical imbalance that might be causing the problem.

MEMORY CHECK

Some of us have a gradual decline in memory and don't even realize it. This questionnaire will help you to determine where you stand on the memory scale.

- Is your memory deteriorating? ____
- Do you find it hard to concentrate and often get confused? ____
- Do you sometimes forget the name of someone you know quite well? ____
- Do you often find you can remember things from the past but forget what you did yesterday? ____
- Do you ever forget what day of the week it is? ____
- Do you ever go looking for something and forget what you are looking for? ____
- Do your friends and family think you're more forgetful than you used to be? ____
- Do you find it hard to add numbers without writing them down? ____
- Do you often experience mental tiredness? ____
- Do you find it hard to concentrate for more than one hour? ____
- Do you often misplace your keys? ____
- Do you frequently repeat yourself? ____
- Do you sometimes forget the point you're trying to make? ____
- Does it take you longer to learn things than it used to? ____

Scoring
   1–5: You don't have a major problem with your memory—but you'll find that supplementing with natural mind and memory boosters will sharpen your memory even more.

6–10: Your memory definitely needs a boost—you are starting to suffer from brain drain. Follow all the diet and supplement recommendations in Chapter 3 and check your stress levels.

11–14: You are experiencing significant memory decline and need to do something about it. As well as following the diet and supplement recommendations in Chapter 3, see a nutritionist who can identify other causes of memory decline, such as a stress hormone imbalance, especially if you also scored high on the stress questionnaire.

CONNECTION CHECK

Check out how "connected" you feel. You may be more alone or isolated than you realize.

- Do you lack a sense of self-worth? ____
- Do you lack enthusiasm? ____
- Are you bored? ____
- Do you feel lonely much of the time or find it difficult to be alone? ____
- Do you feel disconnected from your local community or your workplace? ____
- Do you lack good friends you can really talk to? ____
- Do you feel different, like the "odd one out"? ____
- Do you lack a sense of purpose or meaning in your life? ____
- Are you unclear about your spiritual values? ____
- Do you find it difficult to receive love from others? ____
- Do you lack a sense of peace and contentment? ____
- Do you seldom have experiences of great joy or love? ____
- Do you seldom feel a connection with nature? ____
- Do you abuse your body with bad diet, drugs, overwork, or lack of rest? ____

Any "Yes" answer indicates some measure of disconnection. Higher scores will reflect an underlying tendency to depression as well. If your mood score seems to correlate with this one, first cover the basics of the mood enhancers in Chapter 6. Then, the advice in Chapter 8 will help you to feel more connected to yourself and others and to develop a sense of meaning and purpose. Consider taking up group activities that promote all of these, such as yoga, t'ai chi, or meditation classes.

Scoring

1–5: You have some degree of disconnection.

6–10: Your level of disconnection is a cause for concern, and you may have a tendency toward depression. Be sure to read Chapter 8 and monitor yourself to make sure the situation doesn't worsen.

11–14: You are experiencing a high degree of disconnection and should reevaluate your life regarding what is important to you. Besides following the advice above, consider seeing a counselor or psychotherapist, or attending a personal development course (see the Resources section).

2

How Your Brain Keeps You High

The brain is a remarkable organ. Weighing a mere three pounds, it has the capacity to hold countless memories and allows us to experience the beauty of music, the ecstasy of love, the thrills of sex, and, for some of us, the bliss of inner peace. It's also the abode of fear, anxiety, and deep depression. Understanding how the brain works will help you to enhance positive experiences and decrease the negative ones. You will also see why some substances knock your brain out of balance, while others make it hum.

Neurotransmitters:
Getting the Message Across

The keys to your brain function are the chemical messengers of mind and mood called *neurotransmitters*. As they whizz around your brain and nervous system, they help determine how you feel.

Trillions of nerve cells, called *neurons*, are scattered throughout the body but are most highly concentrated in the brain. Connecting to one another via branches called *dendrites*, they link together like interconnecting highways. Neurotransmitters deliver messages from one neuron to the next. The "sending" neuron produces the neurotransmitter, propelling it toward the "receiving" neuron, across a small gap called a *synapse*. There it attaches to its specific receptor site, just like a key fitting into a lock. When it fits, the message is delivered—that is, the receptor is activated. An electrical signal then travels along the dendrites until it reaches the next synapse or road junction, where it triggers the release of more neurotransmitters.

Once a neurotransmitter has delivered its message, it is released from the receptor site and returns to the synapse. It might then be taken up once again into the neuron that sent it, where it can be used again, or it might be broken down and destroyed.

Each neuron, on average, makes more than 1,000 synaptic connections with other neurons. In total, there may be between 100 trillion and a quadrillion synapses in the brain. Moreover, these synapses are not random but form patterns that give rise to what are called *circuits* in the brain. These form the basis of behavior and of mental life. How you think and feel—your mood, alertness, level of relaxation, and the state of your memory—is affected by the fine-tuned activity of these circuits, which are controlled by the interplay of the various neurotransmitters.

One of the most awe-inspiring mysteries of brain science is how neuronal activity within circuits gives rise to behavior and, even, consciousness. We don't mean to oversimplify by saying that the level of any one neurotransmitter in the brain, such as serotonin, is the only influence on mood and behavior. There is, in fact, a delicately balanced system in place involving our genetic makeup, environmental influences, memories, and neuronal health. We can, however, influence neuronal activity by supplying the right nutrients to make them work optimally, including the raw materials to produce the neurotransmitters. To put it simply: enough of the happy ones make you feel high, while deficiency will leave you feeling unmotivated or tired.

While there are hundreds of neurotransmitters, the following are the main players:

- **GABA** (gamma-aminobutyric acid) is the "cool" neurotransmitter, relaxing you and calming you down after stress.

- **Catecholamines:** The Energizers or Stimulants
  - **Adrenaline** (also called *epinephrine*) is the "motivator," stimulating you and helping you respond to stress.
  - **Dopamine** and **noradrenaline** (also called *norepinephrine*) are the "feel-good" neurotransmitters, making you feel energized and in control.
- **Endorphins** promote "bliss," giving you a sense of euphoria.
- **Acetylcholine** is the "brainy" neurotransmitter, improving memory and mental alertness.
- **Tryptamines:** The "Connection" Neurotransmitters
  - **Serotonin** is the "happy" neurotransmitter, improving your mood and banishing the blues.
  - **Melatonin** helps to keep you in tune with the cycles of nature, regulating your inner clock for day and night, and responds to seasonal shifts.
  - **DMT (dimethyltryptamine)** helps you see "the big picture."

Below is a detailed description of what each of these neurotransmitters does, and what happens when you are deficient.

1. *GABA* (gamma-aminobutyric acid), an inhibitory neurotransmitter, is associated with relaxation. It has a dampening effect on the central nervous system and controls the release of dopamine in the reward center of the brain. A prime example of a GABA-enhancing drug is the tranquilizer Valium. Adequate levels of GABA lead to emotional tranquillity, while low levels of GABA are associated with anxiety, tension, and insomnia.

2. *Adrenaline* is associated with motivation, drive, energy, stimulation, and the stress response. Produced by the adrenal glands, it is also classified as a hormone—which is a chemical messenger produced by the glands of the endocrine system. The hormonal system, while functioning at a much slower pace than the nervous system, works with the nervous system to maintain internal balance and harmony. The adrenal glands are the core of the endocrine system's stress response. They produce about forty hormones, responsible for many bodily functions. Two of their most important hor-

mones, adrenaline and cortisol, are responsible for the "fight or flight" response that controls how we deal with stress. This is explained in detail in Chapter 4.

3. *Dopamine* and *noradrenaline* are associated with pleasure, motivation, alertness, concentration, and euphoria. While both adrenaline and noradrenaline are raised by stress, noradrenaline levels tend to be higher in "positive" stress states including sex, being "in love," exercise, dancing, and listening to music. Both dopamine and noradrenaline are made from the amino acid tyrosine and are classified as catecholamines (see Figure 1 on page 24). Dopamine appears to be the primary neurotransmitter of reward, through the dopamine receptors located in a small area of the brain called the *nucleus accumbens*. This is part of the limbic system, which governs emotions. Under stress, we release a hundred times more dopamine than we do in a normal resting state. For details, see Chapter 5.

Adequate levels of dopamine allow you to focus, to complete tasks, to feel energized and motivated, and to experience pleasure. Low levels are associated with depression, lack of concentration, poor motivation, and difficulty initiating and/or completing tasks.

4. *Endorphins* are the popular term for substances known as "opiate peptides," which include enkephalins and dynorphins. These are associated with pleasure, orgasm, euphoria, and pain relief. Endorphins are the brain's own natural opiates: they bind to a specific opiate receptor, reducing pain and promoting mild euphoria, such as "runner's high." The opiates morphine and codeine are actually found in normal cerebrospinal fluid that surrounds the brain and spinal cord.

Low levels of endorphins are associated with physical and emotional pain, addiction, and risk-taking behaviors.

5. *Acetylcholine* is associated with memory, mental alertness, learning ability, and concentration. Deficiency can lead to memory loss, depression, mood disorders, and possibly even Alzheimer's disease. It is also the neurotransmitter at all nerve-muscle cell junctions that allows skeletal muscles to contract, controlling movement, coordination, and muscle tone. Adequate levels of acetylcholine provide mental alertness and agility, while low levels

of acetylcholine are associated with poor learning, memory loss, poor concentration, difficulty visualizing, lack of dreaming, and dry mouth.

6. *Serotonin* is associated with mood, sleep patterns, dreaming, and visions. It influences many physiological functions, including blood pressure, digestion, body temperature, and pain sensation. Serotonin also affects mood, as well as circadian rhythm, the body's response to the cycles of day and night.

Adequate levels of serotonin provide emotional and social stability, while low levels of serotonin are associated with depression; anxiety; premenstrual syndrome (PMS); increased sexual drive; carbohydrate cravings; sleep disturbances; increased sensitivity to pain; emotional volatility, including violent behavior against self and others; obsessive thinking; alcohol and drug abuse; and suicide.

7. *Melatonin* also acts as an antidepressant with antiaging properties. However, its main role seems to be keeping you "in sync" with the rhythms of nature. Melatonin harmonizes brain function with day and night, through its sensitivity to light. **Note:** It can help the brain to adjust to a new time zone, thereby avoiding jet lag, if taken as a supplement at bedtime. (Take 1 mg for each hour time difference the first night, then half that amount on the second night, half again on the third night, until you are back in sync.)

8. *DMT* (**dimethyltryptamine**) is thought to be produced primarily in the pineal gland, along with melatonin. It is associated with peak experiences and major insights. It is thought to be released at birth, facilitating an infant's transition from womb to world, and at death, facilitating the transition from this realm of existence to the next.

You Are What You Eat

These are the main players in the orchestra of your brain and nervous system. The secret to being naturally high is finding the right balance of substances and circumstances that get them playing in perfect harmony. One basic principle here is that you are what you eat.

Neurotransmitters are made from amino acids, which come from the protein that we eat. There are eight essential amino acids. From these eight, we can make all the other amino acids that our brains and bodies need, and from these we make the neurotransmitters. In Figure 1 below, you can see how the neurotransmitter serotonin is made from the amino acid trypto-

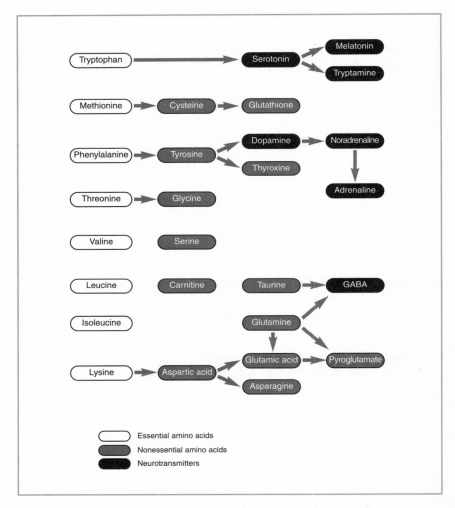

Figure 1. Family tree of neurotransmitters made from amino acids. Arrows show conversions related to neurotransmitter production. There are many others that occur but have been omitted for simplicity.

phan. We know that serotonin, provided by tryptophan-rich foods, such as turkey or milk, can improve your mood.

This was shown very clearly by an experiment carried out at Oxford University's Department of Psychiatry. Eight women were given a diet devoid of tryptophan. Within a mere eight hours, most of them started to feel more depressed. When tryptophan was added to their diet—and without their knowledge—their mood improved.

The popular antidepressant drugs fluoxetine (Prozac) and sertraline (Zoloft) are called *selective serotonin reuptake inhibitors,* or *SSRIs.* When we block the neurons' reuptake of serotonin, there is more of the neurotransmitter available, resulting in a better mood. For more information, see Chapter 6.

The Starbucks Effect

Mind-altering substances work by changing the balance of neurotransmitters. To better understand how this happens, let's take a look at your response to a cup of coffee:

- Within minutes, you experience increased alertness and heightened focus.
- Your mood may improve, and your memory may seem a bit sharper.
- You might also begin to feel jittery.
- You may soon have the urge to urinate. (Coffee is a diuretic.)
- In an hour or two, you might notice yourself feeling down, foggy, and drowsy, and even irritable or cranky. You will probably start to crave another cup of coffee.

This is what is going on in your brain: The stimulant compounds in coffee—caffeine, theobromine, and theophylline—cause the excessive release of the neurotransmitter dopamine. Dopamine is then turned into adrenaline and noradrenaline. This trio of stimulating neurotransmitters makes you feeling motivated and energized.

At the same time, adrenaline causes glucose, or blood sugar, to be released into your system, stimulating both mind and body, much like a hit of any source of sugary food, such as a doughnut. Adrenaline also acts as a diuretic, increasing the need to urinate.

But the effects don't end there. In an hour or two, it's as if you never had that cup of coffee—and you're likely to want another. Unfortunately, the next one is unlikely to provide the same kick. Too frequent consumption will lead to a decreased response known as *tolerance*.

Now you're hooked. If you don't get your morning fix of coffee you may feel tired and cranky. You may even develop a headache. This is due to *withdrawal*, the negative symptoms that *appear* when a substance is *stopped*, and *disappear* when it is *reinstated*. Soon you are in the grip of a compulsive need for more—the curse of the substances that we use to get high, from coffee to cocaine and cigarettes to alcohol. What's worse is that the more you are addicted to a substance, the less benefit you get from it.

Why Doesn't It Last?
The Brain's Ups and Downs

Why do you need more and more caffeine, nicotine, or alcohol to get the same effect? Remember the kick from your first cigarette, cup of coffee, or drink of alcohol? For some, it's the first snort of cocaine or hit of Ecstasy. Have you ever wondered why you don't experience that same high anymore?

The brain has a set of negative feedback mechanisms whose goal is to prevent us from being too stimulated for too long. When we boost our feel-good neurotransmitters, the released dopamine causes a feeling of well-being. However, in response, the receptors gradually shut down, deflating our high.

A key concept in the body and brain, as in all of nature, is *balance*. Much as a thermostat keeps our home at a desired temperature, the body has ways of maintaining a state of equilibrium. The body's self-regulation process, then, makes it impossible for us to gain any long-term benefit from the use of stimulants. Herein lies the rub. In response to an increase in the amount of available neurotransmitter, such as dopamine, there is a "down-regulation" of the receptor sites. To make the neuron less responsive, some receptor sites shut down. Consequently, you need more of the stimulant—caffeine, nicotine, cocaine, or whatever—to release dopamine into the synapses and get the message across.

As a result, you feel tired, unmotivated, and in need of another hit of stimulant, and in increasing amounts. No longer will that regular cup of coffee (around 100 mg of caffeine) give you the kick-start. Now you require a double espresso (around 400 mg), perhaps with a cigarette thrown in, or even a mochaccino (chocolate plus coffee, providing two different stimulants).

Continue along this slippery path for long enough and the effects of the stimulant become nothing like they used to be. No longer does that cup of coffee give you a rush of energy. Now all it does is relieve your ever-increasing fatigue. You need coffee just to feel normal! You've been trying to cheat the system, and it's fighting back. Crime, as far as falsely stimulating your neurotransmitters is concerned, doesn't pay.

Unfortunately, by the time you realize this and stop using the substance, your body's chemistry doesn't give you an unconditional pardon. Instead, it punishes you with withdrawal. In effect, the withdrawal period is the time it takes from the moment you quit using stimulants until your neurons "upregulate" to resensitize once more to normal stimulation. In the case of caffeine, this is only a matter of days. For nicotine or heroin, this process can take weeks.

Essential Fats: Getting the Message

So far we've been talking about the way neurotransmitters deliver messages. Now let's look more closely at how the neurons receive the message. The receptor sites are found in the insulating layer, the myelin sheath, which is roughly 75 percent fat. Thus, to get the message, you need a good supply of the same essential fatty acids (EFAs) that form the sheath. Another component is the phospholipids, which help the message travel smoothly along the nerve. You'll find out about these in detail in Chapter 3.

THREE WAYS TO GET YOUR BRAIN COMMUNICATING

You now know that there are three possible ways to influence or enhance your neurotransmitter balance and thereby enhance your mind and mood.

1. *Sufficient neurotransmitters.*
   You must supply your brain with enough nutrients (in most cases, amino acids) to make the neurotransmitters you need. As we saw in the case above, a tryptophan-poor diet can lead to depression, which can be reversed by consuming the right foods or supplementing with either L-tryptophan or its cousin, 5-hydroxytryptophan (5-HTP).

2. *Better reception.*
   To keep your brain receptors in tip-top shape, you must take enough EFAs, especially omega-3s, and phospholipids, which are explained in greater detail in the next chapter. Unstable moods and problems with memory and cognition may be due to an inadequate supply of these oils. Eat more fish, and add lecithin granules, which are high in phospholipids.

3. *Better transmission and reception.*
   Using and abusing various substances lead the body to compensate by downregulation. This makes it harder to quit an addictive substance.

Congratulations—you've now completed your introduction to brain chemistry. You saw how the common substances we use to give us a short-term boost can lead to burnout through tolerance, addiction, and withdrawal. The secret to being naturally high is to tune up your neurotransmitters using specific natural, healthy, and nonaddictive nutrients and herbs.

3

Natural High Basics

You are what you eat.
R. J. CRUMBE

Let food be your medicine.
HIPPOCRATES

Food as Fuel

If you want to be naturally high, you must begin with the best possible raw materials to feed both your body and mind. Many people in North America fail this basic first step because our Standard American Diet (SAD for short!) is anything but nourishing. Ironically, we are overfed and under-nourished. With a diet consisting of processed food that is nearly devoid of nutrient value, high in chemicals, salt, and, above all, sugar, it's amazing that our bodies can eke out the basic minimum requirements. Often, they don't. We need a steady supply of high-quality fuel (food) for our engines (bodies and brains) in order to function on all cylinders.

In our practices we have seen depressed, low-energy, foggy-brained adults who were not, as they had been erroneously told, in need of Prozac, but simply needed a consistent supply of "real food" to get their brains and bodies going. Haven't there been times when you found yourself feeling tired, irritable, and unable to think straight, and overwhelmed with all that you had to do when you realize that you'd skipped a meal? Within minutes

29

of eating a carrot, or a piece of cheese, everything changes—the world becomes a better place, and those tasks are no longer insurmountable. The problem was simply low blood sugar: your poor brain was running on empty! More on this issue in the next chapter. Suffice it to say, you need to maintain your blood-sugar level as a basic step to feeling consistently high.

The next step is to choose the highest-quality food possible to help keep your neurotransmitters in balance.

There is scientific proof that if you follow the principles of optimum nutrition, you can:

- Improve your mood.
- Increase your mental and physical stamina.
- Enhance your concentration, memory, and overall mental ability.
- Reduce your stress level.

In this chapter, we'll be looking at each of the various nutrients from the fuel-supplying carbohydrates to the building-block proteins and fats to the catalysts and cofactors, vitamins and minerals. We'll finish with a list of the basics that will get you—and keep you—high.

Running on Carbohydrates

The main fuel for all body cells, including brain cells, is glucose, or blood sugar. Most carbohydrates—bread, cereals, fruits, and vegetables—break down into this simple sugar during digestion. Despite its weight of only 3 pounds, the brain is the most sugar-hungry organ of the body, consuming up to 50 percent of ingested glucose. This does not mean that you should eat more sugar to enhance your brain power! Quite the opposite. The quick-release sugars—found in white flour, candy, cookies, and fruit juices—will lead only to the "sugar blues."

We measure how quickly a specific food is turned into glucose by means of the Glycemic Index (GI). To determine the GI of a particular food, a measured portion is fed to participants, whose blood is analyzed over the course of several hours. The higher the GI of the food, the faster the resultant rise in blood sugar will be after eating it. As your blood sugar goes higher, more insulin is secreted to cope with the sugar. Insulin removes sugar and stores it as fat and glycogen. High-glycemic foods, such as dough-nuts and candy, cause insulin to spike rapidly and excessively. This causes your blood-glucose levels to drop, making you feel weak, lightheaded, and even cranky.

The top brain-fuel foods, however, are "slow-release" carbohydrates—those that gradually and consistently release their energy-giving glucose into the bloodstream, allowing for more stable blood-glucose levels. Some low GI "good guys" include complex carbohydrates, such as whole, unre-fined grains, found in whole-grain bread and whole-wheat pasta. Some fruits, like apples and pears, have a low GI, while others, such as raisins and bananas, have much higher GIs. Almost all vegetables are slow-releasing. While this index can be very useful in helping us avoid high-glycemic vil-lains, it's important to factor in a food's nutritional component along with its GI. While carrots, raisins, and bananas are relatively high on the GI, we certainly don't recommend that you avoid these nutritious and delicious foods. Certainly, no one ever got too fat from eating these foods. So defer to your common sense and use the GI as a guide, not your bible!

Another way to slow the release of carbohydrates is to combine them with protein. For example, pair a salmon steak with brown basmati rice, chicken with boiled new potatoes, or, if you're vegetarian, tofu with whole-wheat pasta.

For an ideal diet, choose the low GI foods that score under 50 on pages 32–35. Eat others sparingly.

The Power of Protein

You can influence how you feel simply by consuming the ideal quantity of protein. Made up of amino acids, protein is the building block of all bodily components, from hair and muscles to enzymes and hormones, as well as the source of neurotransmitters. The quality of a protein is determined by its balance of amino acids. Higher-quality protein is better absorbed and more efficiently utilized, so you will need less of it to be optimally nourished.

Our bodies require twenty-three different amino acids for proper function, nine of them "essential"—lysine, tryptophane, methionine, valine,

The Complete Glycemic Index (GI) of Foods
(For an ideal diet, choose the low
GI foods that score under 50.)

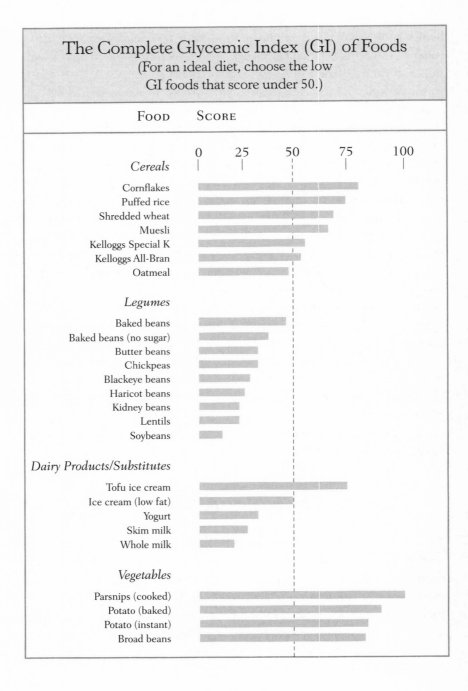

FOOD	SCORE

Cereals

Cornflakes
Puffed rice
Shredded wheat
Muesli
Kelloggs Special K
Kelloggs All-Bran
Oatmeal

Legumes

Baked beans
Baked beans (no sugar)
Butter beans
Chickpeas
Blackeye beans
Haricot beans
Kidney beans
Lentils
Soybeans

Dairy Products/Substitutes

Tofu ice cream
Ice cream (low fat)
Yogurt
Skim milk
Whole milk

Vegetables

Parsnips (cooked)
Potato (baked)
Potato (instant)
Broad beans

FOOD	SCORE

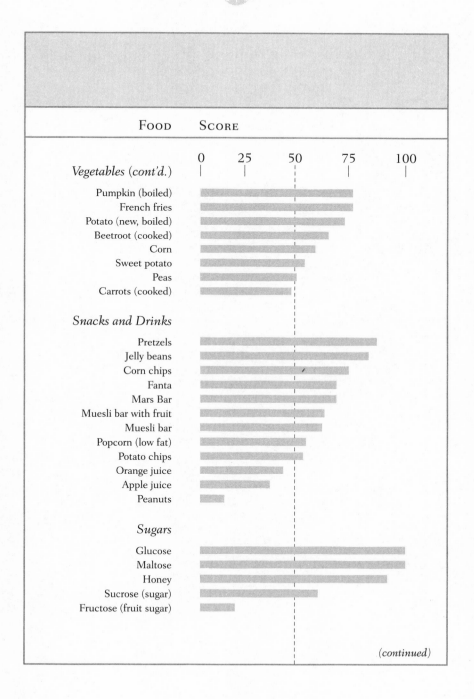

Vegetables (cont'd.)

	0	25	50	75	100

Pumpkin (boiled)
French fries
Potato (new, boiled)
Beetroot (cooked)
Corn
Sweet potato
Peas
Carrots (cooked)

Snacks and Drinks

Pretzels
Jelly beans
Corn chips
Fanta
Mars Bar
Muesli bar with fruit
Muesli bar
Popcorn (low fat)
Potato chips
Orange juice
Apple juice
Peanuts

Sugars

Glucose
Maltose
Honey
Sucrose (sugar)
Fructose (fruit sugar)

(continued)

The Complete Glycemic Index (GI) of Foods
(For an ideal diet, choose the low GI foods that score under 50.)

FOOD	SCORE

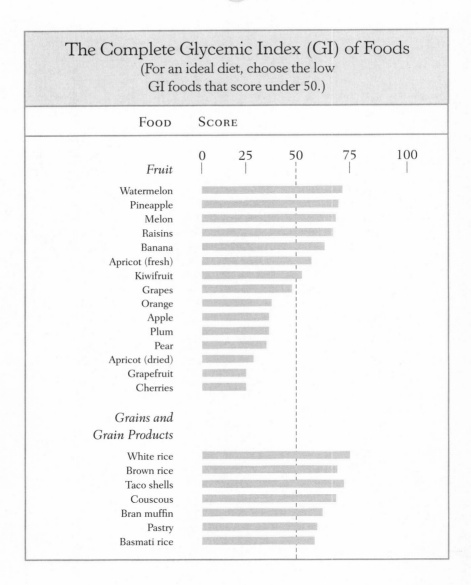

Fruit

Food	Approx. Score
Watermelon	~72
Pineapple	~66
Melon	~65
Raisins	~64
Banana	~62
Apricot (fresh)	~57
Kiwifruit	~52
Grapes	~46
Orange	~44
Apple	~38
Plum	~38
Pear	~37
Apricot (dried)	~30
Grapefruit	~25
Cherries	~22

Grains and
Grain Products

Food	Approx. Score
White rice	~72
Brown rice	~66
Taco shells	~68
Couscous	~65
Bran muffin	~60
Pastry	~59
Basmati rice	~58

Food	Score

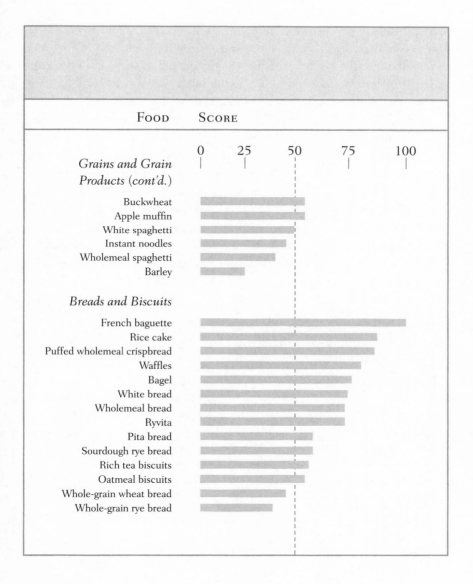

Grains and Grain Products (cont'd.)

	0 25 50 75 100
Buckwheat	
Apple muffin	
White spaghetti	
Instant noodles	
Wholemeal spaghetti	
Barley	

Breads and Biscuits

| French baguette |
| Rice cake |
| Puffed wholemeal crispbread |
| Waffles |
| Bagel |
| White bread |
| Wholemeal bread |
| Ryvita |
| Pita bread |
| Sourdough rye bread |
| Rich tea biscuits |
| Oatmeal biscuits |
| Whole-grain wheat bread |
| Whole-grain rye bread |

leucine, isoleucine, histidine, threonine, and phenylalanine. Because our bodies cannot make them, they must be derived from our diet. We are able to manufacture the remaining amino acids, though at the cost of diverting precious materials and energy. So it's still better to ingest as large a variety of amino acids as possible, even the so-called nonessential ones.

Meat, fish, chicken, poultry, cheese, milk, and eggs are considered complete proteins, since they contain the essential amino acids and in sufficient amounts. Plants can be sources of protein, too, but the only complete one is soy. You can, however, combine plant-based proteins that are missing one or two amino acids, to create a complete protein; for example, whole grains, nuts, or seeds with a serving of beans, or rice and beans.

The quality of a protein source can be measured according to its net protein usability (NPU)—or the balance of its amino acids. The table below shows some examples of high-quality protein choices, either alone or in

Packed with Protein: The Top 24

Food	Percentage of Calories as Protein	How Much for 2–4 Ounces of Protein	Protein Quality (NPU)
Grains/Legumes			
Quinoa	16	3½ oz/1 cup dry weight	Excellent
Tofu	40	10 oz/1 packet	Reasonable
Corn	4	1 lb 2 oz/3 cups cooked weight	Reasonable
Brown rice	5	14 oz/3 cups cooked weight	Excellent
Chickpeas	22	4 oz/0.66 cup cooked weight	Reasonable
Lentils	28	3 oz/1 cup cooked weight	Reasonable

Fish/Meat

Tuna, canned	61	3 oz/1 small can	Excellent
Cod	60	1¼ oz/1 very small piece	Excellent
Salmon	50	3½ oz/1 very small piece	Excellent
Sardines	49	3½ oz/1 grilled	Excellent
Chicken	63	2½ oz/1 small roasted breast	Excellent

Nuts/Seeds

Sunflower seeds	15	6½ oz/1 cup	Reasonable
Pumpkin seeds	21	2½ oz/0.5 cup	Reasonable
Cashew nuts	12	4 oz/1 cup	Reasonable
Almonds	13	4 oz/1 cup	Reasonable

Eggs/Dairy

Eggs	34	4 oz/2 medium	Excellent
Yogurt, natural	22	1 lb/3 small containers	Excellent
Cottage cheese	49	4½ oz/1 small container	Excellent

Vegetables

Peas, frozen	26	9 oz/2 cups	Reasonable
Other beans	20	7 oz/2 cups	Reasonable
Broccoli	50	1½ oz/0.5 cup	Reasonable
Spinach	49	1½ oz/0.66 cup	Reasonable

Combinations

Lentils and rice	18	4½ oz/small cup dry weight	Excellent
Beans and rice	15	4½ oz/small cup dry weight	Excellent

combination. It also shows what portion size you need to consume to get about an ounce of protein per serving. A man needs to eat the equivalent of three to four of the indicated servings, while a woman needs to eat two to three.

A typical allotment of protein for a man might therefore include an egg for breakfast, a 7-ounce salmon steak for lunch, and a serving of beans with dinner.

For a vegetarian, a typical day might include a small container of yogurt and a heaping tablespoon of seeds on an oat-based cereal for breakfast, and a 9.5-ounce serving of tofu, and vegetable stir-fry, served with either a cup of quinoa or a serving of beans with rice as part of dinner.

Vegetarians need to eat "seed" foods—that is, foods that would grow if you planted them. These include seeds, nuts, beans, lentils, peas, corn, or the germ of grains such as wheat or oat. "Flower" foods, such as broccoli or cauliflower, are also relatively rich in protein. Lentils or beans plus brown rice provide an excellent source of complete protein.

Caution: Too much protein intake encourages fat storage and can also lead to ketosis, in which muscle tissue is broken down to produce glucose for the brain. This is the principle behind the Atkins Diet which, carried beyond his suggested initial two weeks, can be unsafe. Excessive protein can also contribute to osteoporosis, kidney disease, and heart disease.

Alpha and Omega:
The Essential Fats for the Brain

Now that you understand the value of essential amino acids derived from protein, let's take a look at essential fatty acids, which are mainly derived from oils, seeds, and fish. Fatty acids are the molecular components of fats and oils. They come in several categories: saturated, monounsaturated, and polyunsaturated. We're going to focus on the healthy polyunsaturated fatty acids from which vital omega-3 and omega-6 fatty acids are derived.

Most people aren't aware that certain fats are vital to health. The essential fatty acids produce hormones called *eicosanoids,* which are necessary for many chemical processes within the body. They stimulate the immune system, fight inflammation, and support the activity of neurotransmitters, including serotonin. In fact, fats comprise 60 percent of the brain, and the essential fats make a big difference in brain cell communication, powerfully affecting mind and mood.

The popularity of very low- to non-fat diets in recent years has actually contributed to a whole host of problems, from premenstrual syndrome (PMS) and infertility to depression and anxiety, and even to premature aging. About 30 percent of the calories in your diet should come from beneficial fat. While the bad fats can be incorporated into the brain, they are not functional and can actually numb your thinking processes and worsen your mood; therefore, it's important to avoid saturated and hydrogenated fats in the forms of meat, dairy products, and junk foods.

For optimal brain function, you need the polyunsaturated oils, the omega-3 and omega-6 essential fatty acids (EFAs), in a ratio of 1:1 and 1:2, respectively. The typical modern diet, though, is usually far too high in omega-6 oils (more like 1:20 to 1:30). The omega-6 oils are found in meats, milk, vegetable oils, seeds (sesame, hemp, sunflower, and pumpkin), and nuts, so getting enough is less of a problem in the average diet. Most of us have to work to ensure our intake of omega-3s, found in flaxseeds and in fish, especially fatty cold-water fish such as mackerel, tuna, and salmon.

For an adequate omega-3 supply, you should have a serving of fatty fish three times a week *or* 1,000 mg of EPA and DHA (combined) daily. If you are a strict vegetarian, you should take a teaspoon of flaxseed oil daily *or* a heaping tablespoon of seeds every day—half flaxseeds, and half sesame, sunflower, hemp, and pumpkin-seed mix, ground up in a coffee grinder to release the nutrients within. To ensure freshness, keep them in a tightly sealed glass jar in the refrigerator. Sprinkle the mixture over cereal or add it to a shake.

You can also buy organic cold-pressed seed oil blends that provide both omega-3 and omega-6 fats, and use in salad dressings or on just-cooked vegetables instead of butter. Don't use these polyunsaturated oils for frying, as this will denature them.

Phospholipids: The Insulation Experts

Another family of "intelligent" fat in your brain, the phospholipids *phosphatidyl choline* and *phosphatidyl serine,* forms the insulating layer, or myelin sheath, that covers all nerve cells. They also enhance your mood and mental performance, protecting against age-related memory decline and Alzheimer's disease.

Although the body can make them, getting extra phospholipids from food is highly beneficial. Egg yolk is the richest source of phospholipids in the average diet. But since egg phobia set in, amid fears that dietary cholesterol was a major cause of heart disease, the average intake of phospholipids dropped dramatically. (The American Heart Association now states that you can eat up to seven eggs a week.) Significantly, cases of Alzheimer's disease have sky-rocketed.

Lecithin is an excellent source of phospholipids and is widely available in health food stores as either granules or capsules. The easiest and cheapest way is to add lecithin to your diet is to sprinkle a tablespoon of lecithin granules or a heaping teaspoon of high-PC lecithin on your cereal or add it to your protein drink in the morning. Or you can take four lecithin capsules providing 1,200 mg each. By the way, lecithin doesn't make you fat. In fact, quite the opposite occurs: it helps your body to metabolize fat.

Which Diet Is Best?

In the past ten years, Americans have reduced their fat intake and increased their carbohydrate intake. Dr. Barry Sears, author of *Mastering the Zone,* believes that this dietary shift to carbohydrates has contributed to the rise in health problems, including weight gain, arthritis, heart disease, and cancer. He recommends that people reduce their carbohydrate intake while increasing their fat and protein intake, in a 40 percent to 30 percent to 30 percent ratio of carbohydrates, proteins, and fats, respectively. While good in many respects, there are concerns about protein intakes as high as 30 percent of calories. This is because high-protein diets are strongly linked to an increased risk of osteoporosis.

We recommend a more tempered balance—50 percent complex carbohydrates, 30 percent "good" fat, and 20 percent good-quality protein. This means reducing your intake of refined carbohydrates and sugar, and instead choosing whole, complex carbohydrates from fresh fruit, vegetables, whole grains, and cereals. We also recommend increasing omega-3 fats from fish and seeds, while reducing saturated fats from butter, fatty meat, margarine, processed foods containing hydrogenated fats, and deep-fried foods. While eggs are a good source of protein, they tend to be very high in saturated fats. Range-fed organic eggs, especially from chickens that are fed a high omega-3 fat diet, eaten boiled or poached, are an excellent source of protein and 'good' fats. Unpasteurized dairy products from a certified dairy that uses no antibiotics or hormones are also a good source of protein, provided you are not allergic to dairy. These whole, unadulterated foods are much healthier for you than intensively reared animal products, and less likely to cause allergic reactions.

If you'd like more information about how to put the 'Natural High Basics' into practice, please read the *Optimum Nutrition Bible* by Patrick Holford (see Resources). This book explains in detail how to revamp your diet to achieve the optimal amounts of fat, protein, and carbohydrate, plus all essential vitamins, minerals, and other nutrients.

Water, Water . . .

Two-thirds of your body, and almost half of your brain, is made up of water, making it vital for optimal brain and body function. With age, your water content decreases, so drinking enough water can slow the aging process. The ideal intake is around eight 8-ounce glasses a day, and more if you live in a hot climate or exercise heavily.

Fruits and vegetables contain around 90 percent water, in a form that is easy for the body to use. (They are also, of course, a great source of vitamins, minerals, and fiber.) In sufficient quantities, they can provide nearly a quart of water, leaving just an extra quart or so to be taken as water or diluted juices, and herbal or fruit teas. We don't recommend alcohol, caffeinated tea, or coffee as sources of fluid intake, since they are diuretics, and flush out water, together with other valuable nutrients.

One way to increase your water intake is to keep a bottle of filtered or spring water on your desk at work. Fill it up in the morning and drink it all by the time you go home.

Mopping Up with Antioxidants

Oxygen is the ultimate "essential"—a few minutes without it and you're dead. We need to breathe it, of course, and "burning" food with oxygen gives our bodies energy.

The trouble is, whenever we make energy, we also make toxic by-products called *free radicals*—a whole bucketful of them a year. And many of us produce far more than this. One puff of a cigarette, for example, lets loose a trillion free radical molecules in the smoker. Exhaust fumes, pollution, fried and browned food, and exposure to the sun can be equally disastrous. Free radicals are the major cause of the aging process. They attack brain cells and are largely responsible for the decline in their number as we age.

How can you keep free radicals at bay? Increase your intake of antioxidants, a family of nutrients with the power to mop them up, and so reverse the aging process. Top antioxidants include prunes, raisins, blueberries, and blackberries. Kale, spinach, strawberries, raspberries, plums, broccoli, and alfalfa sprouts are close seconds.

Make sure your daily supplement program contains significant quantities of antioxidants, especially if you are older, live in a polluted city, or have any other unavoidable exposure. A comprehensive antioxidant supplement, together with a good multivitamin and mineral tablet, is the best way to go. Each works in its own way, and they work together synergistically. Most high-quality supplement companies produce combination formulas with the following nutrients: vitamin A, beta-carotene, vitamin E, vitamin C, zinc, selenium, glutathione, and cysteine, plus plant-based antioxidants such as anthocyanidins from a source such as bilberry or Pycnogenol.

Essential Cofactors: Vitamins and Minerals

Vitamins and minerals can work real wonders in the brain, where they act as cofactors, or chemical helpers, in the production of neurotransmitters. B vitamins, for instance, can protect you from depression, anxiety, stress, confusion, fatigue, mental dullness, and emotional fragility and can even boost IQ. The minerals magnesium (Mg), iron (Fe), zinc (Zn), manganese (Mn), and chromium (Cr), plus antioxidant nutrients, especially vitamin C, are also vital for brain power and health.

These vital vitamins and minerals are found mostly in whole and "live" food, the fresher the better, and organically grown whenever possible. Whole foods grow in the ground or on trees—they are natural and have undergone little or no processing. They include beans, lentils, seeds, nuts, whole grains such as brown rice, whole-wheat bread or pasta, as well as fresh fruit, vegetables, fish, meat, and eggs. Seeds are especially rich in minerals such as calcium, magnesium, zinc, and iron, as well as in fiber.

The fresh stuff isn't the whole story, though. To achieve optimum health and nutrition, you need to "eat right *and* take a multivitamin," as a recent headline in the *New England Journal of Medicine* editorial put it: "The evidence suggests that people who take such supplements and their children are healthier." A good, high-strength multivitamin plus 1–3 grams of vitamin C a day is your insurance policy for a natural high.

Unconvinced of their power? Consider this research. Ninety students were assigned to one of three groups: one received a multivitamin and mineral supplement; the second, an identical-looking placebo; and the third, nothing. After seven months, the IQ of those taking the supplements had increased by a staggering nine points! A five-point increase would get half the learning disabled children out of special schools and back to normal schooling.

Natural High Basics

- Make sure most of your diet is made up of whole foods and fresh foods.

- Eat three servings a day of top-quality protein foods—fish, poultry, lean meat (free range), egg, soy, or combinations of beans, lentils, and grains.
- Avoid hydrogenated fats and reduce your intake of saturated fats from meat, dairy produce, and junk food.
- Combine protein with carbohydrates.
- Choose low-GI carbohydrates such as whole grains, vegetables, and most fruits, and avoid sugar and refined foods.
- Eat fish three times a week, or take fish-oil supplements.
- Use cold-pressed seed oils on salad dressings.
- Have a heaping tablespoon of ground seeds every day.
- Drink at least a quart of water, if not two, a day, either pure or in diluted juices and herbal or fruit teas.
- Minimize your intake of tea, coffee, and alcohol.
- Eat lots of antioxidant-rich fruits and vegetables—at least five servings a day.
- Take these supplements:
  - A high-potency multivitamin and mineral formula.
  - 1–3 g of vitamin C.
  - An antioxidant formula.
  - Essential fatty acids.

High-Potency Multivitamin and Mineral Formula

A good multivitamin and mineral should provide, at least, the following:

Vitamin A: 20,000 IU total (606 mcg)
[10,000 IU (3,030 mcg) from retinol;
10,000 IU (18 mg) from beta-carotene]
Vitamin D: 100 IU (5mcg)
Vitamin E: 100 IU (67 mg)
Vitamin C: 200 mg

Vitamin B_1 (thiamine): 25 mg
Vitamin B_2 (riboflavin): 25 mg
Vitamin B_3 (niacin/niacinamide): 50 mg
Vitamin B_6: 50 mg
Folic acid: 266 mcg
Vitamin B_{12}: 10 mcg
Biotin: 50 mcg
Pantothenic acid: 50 mg
Coenzyme Q: 20 mg

MINERALS

Calcium: 333 mg
Magnesium: 200 mg
Iron: 10 mg
Zinc (citrate): 10 mg
Iodine: 30 mcg
Copper: 50 mcg
Manganese: 5 mg
Chromium: 100 mcg
Selenium: 100 mcg
Molybdenum: 30 mcg

Part Two

NATURAL ALTERNATIVES

4

Stress Busters

The Stress Cycle

Welcome to life in the twenty-first century where daily stress is so pervasive it seems to be a way of life. We feel pressured to keep up with jobs, family, and the myriad responsibilities of everyday life. Hardly a moment goes by when we are not subject to some form of stress. Many of us end up anxious, depressed, and exhausted—the price we pay for our complex lifestyles. Understanding stress and finding ways of dealing with it effectively are key to living on a natural high. We'll be looking at how stress affects our minds and bodies, as well as at some of the common substances we use to deal with it—even though they are ineffective in the long run. We'll examine the natural antistressors that *do* work, and you'll even see how stress can be turned to your advantage.

Here's a scene that you may be able to relate to (substitute your spouse, your elderly neighbor, or your precious Siamese cat):

It's Monday morning, and you have just enough time to drop your daughter at school and get to work in time for an important meeting. Just as you're both ready to leave the house, she complains of a tummy ache. She does look a bit flushed, so you stop and take her temperature. She has a fever, and you know you can't send her to school. Your mind races: "Should I stay home with her? Can I get a sitter? If not, what do I do about work?"

You have suddenly become a victim of forces beyond your control, pulling you in two directions at once and creating a one-way ticket to stress that wreaks havoc on body and mind.

THE ANATOMY OF STRESS

We need a certain amount of stress to keep us motivated. But when it takes over our lives, it can hurt us. How did you score on the stress questionnaire on page 13? If you didn't take it yet, now is your chance.

Why do we have such a strong reaction to stress? Our particular stressors may be modern, but the stress response is ancient. It mobilizes the body's "fight or flight" response, our built-in mode for coping with emergencies. It increases breathing and heart rate, elevates blood pressure, and raises blood-sugar levels, preparing the body for either self-defense or escape. It worked fine when we were running from fierce predators at the dawn of human existence. However, as much as we'd like to, we can't run from our boss, our stalled car, or the ringing telephone. So, unlike our ancestors, we have no way of burning off this excess energy. In fact, animals in the wild will actually go through a series of movements that disperse the energy and complete the stress cycle right away. We don't, so it stays inside us. Psychologist Peter Levine does an excellent job of exploring this concept in his book *Waking the Tiger*.

On top of this physical burden, we store mental images of traumatic events for years later. These can pop up in our memories at any time in response to similar events, or even at random moments. Then, our minds and bodies react exactly as if the incident were occurring right then—yielding the stress response and anxiety all over again. Some of our problems really are in our minds!

IT'S ALL IN YOUR HEAD

. . . there is nothing either good or bad but thinking makes it so.
HAMLET, ACT 2, SCENE 2

Shakespeare had a point. The truth is, unless your house burns down or someone dies, most stresses are not disasters. Thinking they are, however, can easily overwhelm you. As we said, the problem doesn't even have to be real or present—it can be in the past or the future, or even, *only* in the mind.

When we worry about an upcoming job interview or a blind date, we may find ourselves with a dry mouth, queasy stomach, or sweaty palms. We might become fidgety, restless, and pace around, or have difficulty falling asleep. Our nerves or anxiety are our *emotional response* to stress. Incidentally, anxiety is not always a bad thing. That feeling of apprehension, the gnawing feeling in the pit of our stomachs that "something is wrong" is a natural warning signal. We have all used it as a motivator at times to study for finals or to pay our bills. When it works overtime, though, it causes problems.

ADDICTED TO STRESS

Adrenaline keeps us going, but after awhile it can become addictive. When the stimulus stops (no deadlines while we are on vacation), we experience adrenaline withdrawal, accompanied by restlessness, vague feelings of unease, and a strong desire to "do something," anything, to restart the stress cycle and get the adrenaline pumping once more. If and when we finally let go, we collapse into a heap—depleted, depressed, and exhausted. We may feel blue or bored. Our "get up and go" has "got up and went." We need, in short, to relax, regroup, and rebuild ourselves.

FIGHT OR FLIGHT—THE STRESS RESPONSE

Nobel Prize winner Dr. Hans Selye, the father of stress research, proposed three stages to this stress response. This "General Adaptation Syndrome"

(GAS) consists of alarm, adaptation, and, finally, exhaustion. His model is useful in helping you see where you are in the stress cycle and what to do about it.

Alarm Stage

When you are first stressed, in the *alarm* phase, the brain signals two tiny almond-shaped adrenal glands, perched on top of the kidneys, to produce stress hormones. There are about forty such hormones, but the most important stress hormones are adrenaline, which is manufactured by the inner core; cortisol; and DHEA (dehydroepiandrosterone). Cortisol and DHEA are produced by the outer shell, or *cortex*. Hence the name "adreno*cortico*steroids."

When we are alarmed, the adrenaline effect kicks in immediately, then wanes, but cortisol keeps on going. Both adrenaline and cortisol give a boost to your blood sugar. In fact, the average "adrenaline rush" experienced by a commuter stuck in traffic can supply enough glucose to keep you running for a mile. The adrenals also release the hormone DHEA, which helps maintain energy and resistance to stress.

As a result of this rapid deployment of adrenaline, cortisol, and DHEA, we have more oxygen and sugar available, push more blood to the brain and muscles, and are instantly more alert. In fact, many people will create stress in their lives just to experience this stimulation. It may be stress, but it's also a high.

Adaptation Stage

When the body needs to continue its defense mechanism beyond the initial "fight or flight" response, it enters the *adaptation* phase. Cortisol and DHEA have a reciprocal relationship, so as cortisol levels go up, DHEA levels fall. We start to feel the effects of long-term stress, with increasing anxiety, fatigue, and mood swings.

Exhaustion Stage

When we become stuck in the stress response, it becomes chronic, and we enter the dangerous territory of the *exhaustion* phase. No longer can we produce the necessary cortisol to respond to stress. Our DHEA levels drop. We become depleted of vitamins, including vitamin C, the B vitamins, and essential minerals such as magnesium. Our energy plummets, and since adrenaline is derived from the "feel-good" neurotransmitter dopamine (see page 22), excess adrenaline demands lead to dopamine deficiency. Consequently, our emotions can take a dive into depression.

The Costs of Stress

The extra energy liberated by adrenal stimulation comes at a high cost. In the short term, stress does the following:

- Suppresses the immune system, increasing the risk of infections.
- Slows down the body's rate of repair.
- Slows down metabolism.
- Robs the body of vital nutrients.

The following physical symptoms may occur:

- Recurring headaches.
- Vague aches and pains.
- Dizziness.
- Heartburn.
- Muscle tension.
- Dry mouth.
- Excessive perspiration.
- Pounding heart.
- Insomnia.
- Fatigue.

In the long term, stress will do the following:

- Promote rapid aging.
- Lead to weight gain.
- Increase the risk of developing osteoporosis, high blood pressure, heart disease, cancer, and digestive problems.

(continued)

On an emotional level, when our brains run out of feel-good chemicals, we experience the following:

- Anxiety, fear, restlessness.
- Irritability, anger.
- Depression.
- Insecurity.
- Loss of libido.
- Impaired memory and concentration.
- Excessive smoking and/or drinking.

BLOOD-SUGAR BLUES

Adrenaline and cortisol activity isn't the only danger when we're heavily stressed. Our blood-sugar, or glucose, levels rise, too, then abruptly fall. This is because both adrenaline and cortisol temporarily release stores of sugar into the bloodstream. You can get the same effect from a stimulant, such as coffee, or by eating sugar. Then there's the rebound, and your blood-sugar level plummets. This is serious, because 20 percent of the body's entire intake of glucose fuels the brain, the first area to suffer when glucose is scarce. A dip in blood sugar may leave you feeling tired, nervous, foggy, irritable, impatient, and temperamental. And to relieve this discomfort, you may reach for a doughnut, cola, or cigarette, and a vicious cycle begins.

The good news is that a proper diet and specific nutrients can break this cycle. First, though, let's look at some of the typical solutions to dealing with stress and why they don't work in the end.

Chemical Coping:
Drink, Downers, and Dope

So much for the body's pharmacopia of beneficial and not-so-beneficial solutions to stress. What about all the chemicals in the cupboard that we take to cope? When we're stressed, irritable, or worried, many of us relax with a drink, a joint, or even a prescribed tranquilizer such as Valium (diazepam) or Xanax (alprazolam). They help take the edge off.

You know how it feels. You've just finished a hard day at the office, and you can't wait to get home. You get on the road only to sit in bumper-to-bumper traffic for the next 40 minutes. You arrive home to an equally harried spouse and two noisy kids, vying for your attention. All you want to do is have a drink and forget about everything. . . . Or you're a student with a paper due, and your computer just wiped out an entire afternoon's work. A joint looks really good to you right now. . . . Or you just found out you owe back taxes, and, while you don't know whose fault it is, you're the one who has to come up with the money. Where is that bottle of Valium?

These scenarios may be realistic—but can we say the same about the solutions? The substances that people so often take to chill out have their share of downsides. Let's see how they work and what those downsides are. They include:

- Alcohol.
- Tranquilizers.
- Cannabis.

As you will see, each of these exerts its relaxing effects by boosting these brain chemicals:

- GABA, the relaxing neurotransmitter.
- Dopamine, the "feel-good" neurotransmitter.
- Endorphins, our natural euphoriant.

ALL LIQUORED UP: ALCOHOL EXAMINED

Humans have enjoyed alcohol for at least 6,000 years of recorded history. Today, alcohol plays a pivotal role in society and in economics, with 2.3 billion alcoholic drinks consumed each week in the United States alone.

What happens when you take a drink? Within minutes, that first glass of the evening begins to loosen you up, to lower your inhibitions, and to put you in a cheery and gregarious mood. This effect is due to the release of dopamine, which stimulates you, quickly followed by endorphins, which make you feel high, and then GABA, which helps you relax. The alcohol also gives your blood sugar a boost. Sounds good, doesn't it? That's why we do it. This pleasant effect usually lasts for an hour or so.

Several drinks later, though, you might notice you're feeling irritable, depressed, or even hostile (or others will). Your thinking and memory may become fuzzy. You could end up unsure of where you are, whom you're with, and why you're there. You might then get sleepy or, on a bad night, pass out.

A "hangover"—nausea, headache, and/or stomach upset—may greet you the following morning. You also may have forgotten much of what happened the night before, a phenomenon known as a "blackout." This can be a serious problem especially if you really abandoned your inhibitions. You may now wonder whether the good time was worth it.

Here are some sobering statistics on alcohol consumption:

- A recent study revealed that hangover-induced absenteeism and poor job performance cost the U.S. economy about $148 billion a year.
- Researchers found that people with hangovers posed a danger to themselves and others long after their blood alcohol levels had returned to normal, suggesting that hangovers could be more insidious than the actual inebriation.
- According to the National Highway Traffic Safety Administration, in the year 2000, 40 percent of all fatal car accidents were alcohol-related (*Los Angeles Times*, Oct. 1, 2001).

SEDATIVES AND TRANQUILIZERS: "MOTHER'S LITTLE HELPERS"

From the early 1900s until the mid-1950s, barbiturates such as phenobarbital and Seconal were the drugs of choice for treating anxiety and insomnia. Unfortunately, they also were associated with thousands of suicides and accidental deaths among both children who took them accidentally and

Why Alcohol Is Bad News

SHORT TERM

- Impaired memory: You're not sure where you left your keys, or your car, or who you flirted with (or more) the night before.
- Blackouts: You can recall nothing due to the toxic by-products of alcohol—the information was not stored.
- Impaired sexual function.
- Inappropriate behavior, dehydration, and accidents—including fatal ones.
- Morning-after hangover.

LONG TERM

- Addiction: Though the stimulation caused by alcohol may feel good initially, the brain seeks internal balance, or *homeostasis*. When you keep pushing the brain to release a neurotransmitter, it responds by "downregulating"—that is, reducing production of that specific chemical. The result is that over time, you will need to drink more to keep getting the same effect.
- Long-term alcohol use can lead to a host of health problems such as gastritis, ulcers, liver problems (including cirrhosis, where scar tissue replaces liver cells), pancreatic disease, and permanent brain and nerve damage.
- Pregnant women who abuse alcohol can seriously damage their unborn infants.
- Causes depletion of neurotransmitters and nutrients.
- During acute alcohol withdrawal, chronic alcoholic patients may suffer convulsions from a life-threatening condition called "the DTs" (delirium tremens). DTs can cause hallucinations, convulsive shaking, and other serious physiological changes.

adults who overdosed on them. Other side effects included widespread abuse and dependency, and chemical incompatibility with other drugs and alcohol. By 1954, these drugs were being replaced by the new, "nonaddictive" meprobamate (Miltown) as the calming agent of choice. It turned out to be as addictive as the old drugs.

The 1960s saw the introduction of the currently popular benzodiazepines: diazepam (Valium), chlordiazepoxide (Librium), clonazepam (Klonopin), and the shorter-acting alprazolam (Xanax) and temazepam (Restoril). In the United States alone, 25 million prescriptions are written annually for these so-called "minor tranquilizers" to treat anxiety and insomnia. Their calming effect is due to their action on the receptors for the inhibitory neurotransmitter GABA (gamma-aminobutyric acid). By increasing GABA activity, the benzodiazepines tend to dull awareness and overall brain activity. In effect, they calm your anxiety but also dull your senses.

Marcy is a case in point. At age thirty-five, Marcy found herself stuck in an unhappy marriage and with a young child. Seeing no escape, she began to take large doses of Valium to shut out the pain. One day, while filling yet another prescription for Marcy, the pharmacist said, "In case you don't know it, you're addicted. Speak to me when you're ready to stop." This was her wake-up call.

In shocked response, she simply stopped the drug cold. She was too ashamed to face the pharmacist, who would have advised a slow withdrawal program under medical supervision. Then, not knowing she was suffering from withdrawal symptoms, she simply, in her words, "went crazy" for the next two months or so while she became accustomed to living without the drug.

Valium had caused Marcy's brain (GABA receptors, to be precise) to downregulate in response to Valium's relaxing action. This led to extreme agitation (withdrawal) when she stopped taking it, which lasted until her brain readjusted itself. "When I finally got my mind back, I decided to leave my husband. I never looked back. Nor did I ever dare take another tranquilizer," declares Marcy, now, at forty-eight, a successful writer and a proud grandmother.

Fortunately for Marcy, her pharmacist said the right thing. However, many people addicted to prescription drugs often go for years, having their prescription refilled in large, impersonal pharmacies, or rotating between several different stores. Harried physicians with little time to really listen to

Downsides of Benzodiazepines

Regular usage will cause:

- Tolerance—after taking benzodiazepines for some time, more is required to get the same effect.
- Forgetfulness, drowsiness, accident-proneness, and social isolation.
- Insomnia.
- Hangover—morning-after fogginess or accidents from an undetected hangover (a leading, hidden contributor to automobile accidents).
- Addiction—must continue to take it just to stay "even."
- Serious withdrawal effects upon quitting, including anxiety, insomnia, irritability, tremors, mental impairment, headaches, and possibly even seizures and death.

patients find it easier to renew a prescription than to deal with someone's symptoms. And the prospect of detoxification is a tough one for either of them to deal with.

Be *very* aware that if you are addicted to tranquilizers, withdrawal must be taken seriously. In fact, withdrawal can prove fatal if not done correctly and under medical supervision. See Chapter 9 for details about how to do this safely and naturally with minimal withdrawal symptoms.

CANNABIS: FROM THE STONE AGE TO THE "STONED" AGE

People in Asian and Middle Eastern countries have used marijuana (*Cannabis sativa*) as an intoxicant for thousands of years. With the birth of Islam, cannabis was embraced as the preferred psychoactive substance, replacing the Judeo-Christian favorite, alcohol. Cannabis was later used in Western medicine for at least two millennia, until the early 1900s, when the use of pharmaceuticals largely replaced herbal medicines. It was finally declared illegal for medical use in the 1930s but continued to be used in subcultures, particularly those of artists and musicians.

Then, during the 1960s and 1970s, cannabis use became integrated with the growing counter-culture movement, turning up in communes, colleges, and wherever young people gathered. Today, cannabis is consumed by 11.2 million Americans over age eleven—including baby-boomers who never stopped using it—making it the most widely used of all illegal drugs.

How does it work? The immediate effects of smoking cannabis are mild euphoria and, often, drowsiness. Research shows that brain receptors respond to cannabis by releasing the feel-good neurotransmitter, dopamine. Cannabis's effects on judgment, coordination, and short-term memory make it inadvisable to drive, to operate heavy machinery, or to try to learn anything new while under its influence. This is due to the high concentration of cannabis receptors in both the *hippocampus,* the part of the brain that controls memory, and the *cerebellum,* the part of the brain that governs motor coordination. Moreover, these effects may actually last longer than those of alcohol.

Up in Smoke: Side Effects

Research on the effects of driving under the influence of cannabis concludes that cannabis-induced impairment persists from four to eight hours—long after the subjective effects have worn off. Ninety-four percent of subjects fail roadside sobriety tests 90 minutes after smoking, while 60 percent fail after 150 minutes. Just as with those from alcohol and tranquilizers, the effects from cannabis use last longer than is easily recognized, resulting in needless accidents.

Researchers have found that daily cannabis users, after several days of abstinence, continue to show subtle but measurable impairment in their mental processing. But it's not clear whether this after-the-fact impairment results from changes in the brain or from the slow, continuous release of marijuana constituents that have been stored in the brain and fatty tissues.

A recent study by Dr. Harrison Pope and colleagues, published in the American Medical Association's *Archives of General Psychiatry,* provided some interesting findings regarding the long-term cognitive effects of cannabis use. The researchers evaluated three groups: past heavy users, who had smoked no more than twelve times in the prior three months; heavy users, who had not stopped; and light users, who had smoked no more than fifty times in their lifetime). After a 28-day abstinence period, the participants were given a neuropsychological test for memory, attention, and verbal ability on Days 0, 1, 7, and 28. Despite impairment detected in the earlier testing sessions, by Day 28, all three groups scored similarly on the test. The conclusion was that the cognitive impairment caused by cannabis was acute only and was reversible once the intake was stopped.

Here's the experience of Gene, a forty-five-year-old, married physical therapist:

> I'd only smoke a hit or two every other day, but I had been doing this for years. I finally stopped smoking marijuana completely eight months ago, and I feel a lot better. My workouts have improved, and my overall energy level is up. When I smoked, I would feel relaxed at first, but after an hour or so, my mood would dip. I'd get cranky and want another hit. The next one wouldn't do it, though, so I gave up trying. The moodiness was probably due to a low blood-sugar reaction—you know, "the munchies." Then, I'd eat, so I put on too much weight.
>
> I finally decided I'd had enough of it all, and just quit. I became really irritable. Not only was I craving a smoke, but I had to handle all kinds of emotional issues that were coming up, things I hadn't ever dealt with. Fortunately, I had some aromatherapy and herbal products that really helped cut the cravings and lift my mood. Eventually, after about six to eight weeks, my moods evened out. Now, if I find myself wanting a joint to relax, I take a whiff of my aromatherapy oil or a dose of kava. Overall, I'm glad to be over the whole thing. Life feels more real to me now. My wife likes me better now, too. She says I'm more emotionally available, more stable, and nicer to be with!

In our own observations, young people who smoke their way through high school (or even earlier) and continue through young adulthood are more likely to have problems. They seem less able to cope with the challenges of everyday life or to be able to plan appropriately for their futures. Their emotional development seems blunted: the marijuana fog may have prevented them from fully experiencing a complete range of emotions and relationships. Stoned on the hero's journey, they miss the passages necessary for growing up and accepting their place in the adult world.

Pitfalls of Pot

Regular usage will cause:

- Impaired coordination, judgment, and short-term memory, which persists for four to eight hours. May result in accidents.
- Mood swings and irritability due to low blood-sugar reaction.
- Blunted emotional development in young people who are chronic users, leading to problems in coping with everyday challenges and planning for the future.
- Throat and lung irritation, as with tobacco.

Relaxing Naturally

We have seen how drink, downers, and dope work by promoting the relaxing neurotransmitter GABA, the feel-good neurotransmitter dopamine, and the endorphins, or euphoriants. However, these substances also can cause an imbalance in neurotransmitter and blood-sugar levels that can get you into all kinds of trouble, from emotional and mental impairment to addiction. There are healthier, natural choices that achieve the same goal, but without the negative effects.

While the ideal is to be free of stress and therefore have no need to use relaxants at all, the reality is that we do get stressed and want to restore balance. This means we need to:

- Balance our blood sugar.
- Promote release of GABA.
- Support the release of dopamine and endorphins.
- Supply the appropriate nutrients to produce them.

Stress depletes the body of vital nutrients. The more stressed we are, the more quickly we become deficient, and the more of these nutrients we need. For example, we need B vitamins for a smoothly running nervous system and for adrenal hormone production. There are also certain minerals that have a relaxing effect on the body and emotions. Following the "Natural High Basics" in Chapter 3 will give you a solid basis on which to experience the full benefit of natural relaxants.

As we have seen, alcohol, cannabis, and tranquilizers affect one or more of these keys to relaxation. As with Marcy and Gene, they create significant rebound or withdrawal effects. The result is a never-ending cycle of stress—but natural relaxants can help you break it.

RELAXING NATURALLY WITH HERBS

Nature has provided us with a number of safe, effective, and nonaddictive compounds that relax body and mind. These herbs are readily available and inexpensive, and most have passed the true test of time. In fact, most of our pharmaceuticals are actually plant-based compounds that have been modified and refined for more specific actions. Unlike drugs that simply attack symptoms, herbs work more subtly to promote the body's natural functions. Still, herbs can have powerful effects on the body, so if you are pregnant or nursing, always consult with a physician before taking any herb.

Herbs are most effective when used as close to their natural form as possible. Extracts of herbs are "standardized" for the so-called "active ingredients." However, herbs contain a variety of compounds that work together synergistically, so utilizing the whole plant is often more effective. When we separate out the "active ingredient," as in the pharmaceutical model, we may be losing a significant portion of the plant's action.

A case in point is kava. Studies of this plant repeatedly find that the best effects are derived from a whole extract, containing not only a combination of the active fat-soluble compounds kavalactones but also other supporting factors that are yet to be studied. The same is true for St. John's wort. Hypericin, long believed to be the active antidepressant ingredient, has recently been upstaged by hyperforin. The whole plant extract may work better than either of these isolated compounds, indicating an internal synergy.

Lastly, concentrating a substance often removes its protective compounds, thus increasing the possibility of side effects, as is the case with the herb ephedra, discussed in Chapter 5. Another remarkable aspect of herbs is that they combine several different healing properties that may act simultaneously on different systems of the body. Thus, kava can both relax muscles and relieve topical pain, while St. John's wort can ease depression while enhancing the immune system.

In Germany, where doctors can prescribe herbal as well as synthetic products, they frequently choose the more benign—and equally effective—herbs to do the job.

The most popular and effective natural relaxants are listed below.

Herbs
- Kava
- Valerian
- Hops
- Passionflower

Amino Acids
- GABA
- Taurine

Let's explore how these substances work and why they are not only effective but also much better for you than alcohol, tranquilizers, or cannabis.

Kava: The Pacific Herb

Kava, or *Piper methysticum,* which means "intoxicating pepper," has been consumed as a social and ceremonial drink by Pacific Islanders for more than 3,000 years. The first description of this tall, lush plant with heart-shaped leaves came to the West from Captain Cook, on his celebrated voyages through the South Seas. To this day, when village elders or others come together for significant meetings, they begin with an elaborate kava ceremony. Kava also is used to welcome visiting dignitaries: Pope Paul, Queen Elizabeth II, and President Lyndon B. Johnson all were treated to a ceremonial drink at one time. A perfect icebreaker, kava eases tension and allows freer communication. It makes you warm and friendly, and as one early writer put so well, "You cannot hate with kava in you." Less formally, it is drunk daily as a mild after-work inebriant in the islands' ubiquitous kava bars or "nakamals." For some colorful kava stories, see Chris Kilham's book *Kava: Medicine Hunting in Paradise.*

The root is used both for the drink and, in dried form, for a relaxing herbal supplement, mostly for export. Currently, kava is used in Europe and increasingly in the United States to counteract stress, anxiety, and insomnia. But kava is turning out to be increasingly popular, as in the South Pacific, simply as a natural high. We will cover that aspect in Chapter 8.

Research shows that kava often works just as well as the benzodiazepines. Unlike these prescription drugs, however, you don't need to keep increasing the dose to get the same effect, there are no withdrawal problems when you stop taking it, and a low daytime dose will relax you without making you sleepy. In fact, kava can actually enhance concentration. Research shows that, on a word recognition test, it improves reaction time and performance.

This makes it easy to use for specific anxiety-producing situations such as a job interview or a final exam, where you want to be both calm and alert. In higher doses, kava is a natural sleep enhancer. Unlike benzodiazepines, though, it does not suppress REM (rapid eye movement, which occurs during dreaming) sleep, essential to our emotional, mental, and physical well-being. And there's no morning hangover, either.

WHY KAVA IS BETTER THAN ALCOHOL   Like alcohol, kava can help you relax and ease social interactions. But, of the two, only kava allows you to maintain a clear mind, with no hangover.

A Tip from Dr. Cass

I will often use kava tincture or oral spray when struggling to meet a deadline: it relaxes my mind and body, and cuts out mental chatter, while keeping me alert and focused. I love using it when I am too wide-awake to go to sleep, especially when traveling through times zones and I know I will need to be up early and well rested. Two capsules, and I'm out like a light. The next morning, I awaken refreshed and ready to go.

Natural Highs

As novelist and travel writer Paul Theroux says in *The Happy Isles of Oceania*:

> *No one ever went haywire and beat up his wife after binging on yanggona [kava]. No one ever staggered home from a night around the kava bowl and thrashed his children, or insulted his boss, or got tattooed, or committed rape. The usual effect after a giggly interval was the staggers and then complete paralysis.*

After the first two hours of use, alcohol can make you nervous and shaky. Kava, in contrast, is calming. One four-week study of patients with anxiety found that participants experienced dramatic improvements in their symptoms after just one week of kava use, with improvement continuing through week four. In the largest (101 participants) and longest (twenty-five weeks) study to date, German researcher H. P. Volz and colleagues demonstrated that kava provided significant relief of anxiety versus the placebo, or "dummy" pill, and with minimal side effects.

HOW KAVA WORKS   Kava actually promotes relaxation in two different ways—by acting on the limbic system, which is the emotional center of the brain, and directly on muscles. The muscle-relaxing effects make it particularly useful in treating headaches, backaches, and other tension-related pain.

The active ingredients are the kavalactones, taken from the powdered lateral roots of the plant. Since they are fat- or lipid-soluble, they don't dissolve in water but form an emulsion of oil and water in the traditional drink.

Kava is selectively cultivated for specific effects: certain combinations of these cultivars are more relaxing, others more stimulating, and still others more intoxicating. These cultivars are prized for their ability to alter consciousness in various ways. They are generally kept for island use while the rest are exported, much as vintners will hold on to their prized vintages.

Kava's specific effect on neurotransmitters is not entirely clear. It appears, though, that in keeping with its relaxant effects, it enhances the receptivity of the brain's GABA receptors. Unlike alcohol, it neither disturbs blood-sugar balance nor reduces endorphin levels.

How Much Should You Take? Kava is available in various forms—tablets, capsules, and tinctures, and even in sprays. The taste is quite strong, so most people prefer tablets or capsules. The recommended daily adult dose is 60–75 mg of kavalactones, taken two to three times daily. This is equivalent to 200–250 mg of standardized extract containing 30 percent kavalactones, 100–150 mg of 55 percent extract, or 100 mg of a 75 percent extract. As a sedative to aid sleep, the dose is two to three times that amount. For getting high and chilling out, the dose is quite individual—somewhere between the relaxing and sedating doses, generally twice the dose used to help you sleep.

All these numbers may be confusing, but remember, herbs are extracted from natural plants, not manufactured, and the markers (kavalactones, in this case) are given as a percentage of the whole extract. Conveniently, most capsules or tablets are in the range of 60–75 mg of kavalactones each. Then, your dose is an individual matter, depending on your own chemistry. Don't be too concerned with the exact numbers. Rather, start with one capsule and observe your response. Then you can adjust accordingly. Another warning: The first time or two after taking kava, some people feel a little groggy, so just in case, start on a weekend or evening when you don't have to be fully alert. After a few doses, your body gets used to the sensation, and you will probably feel wonderfully relaxed but alert. Of course, if you are using it to zone out, just let it happen.

The tinctures are rather bitter, an acquired taste. They will also numb the inside of your mouth for the first few minutes. An advantage to tinctures is the rapid onset. Taken straight, the liquid is quickly absorbed in the mouth and into the bloodstream before you even swallow. If you prefer, you can take the tincture in fruit juice to cover the taste.

Kava Safety Taken in these typical doses, kava has only mild side effects—occasional skin rashes in sensitive individuals, headache, or mild stomach upset. Chronic high-dose use on the islands (500–2,500 mg of kavalactones every day for years at a time) will sometimes cause a scaly yellow skin rash called "kava dermopathy." It disappears after intake of the herb is stopped.

Despite its excellent past safety record, kava has recently come under the scrutiny of the United States Food and Drug Administration (FDA), which is acting on reports from Europe that kava may damage the liver. Based on these reports, the U.K. has withdrawn sales of kava products pending further investigation. Closer examination of the German and U.S. reports reveals that the vast majority of cases involved the concomitant use of hepatotoxic (liver) drugs and/or alcohol. Furthermore, a clinical study from Duke University showed no adverse effects from kava on the liver. The fact is, you are far likelier to suffer from liver damage by taking the prescription antianxiety drug Valium, yet it is taken by millions daily with little question—and with no major adverse publicity. The over-the-counter pain medication acetaminophen (Tylenol) also has a high incidence of liver toxicity, responsible for 141 deaths in the United States in 1999 and the leading cause of liver failure in Western countries.

Based on the limited information made available to date, we recommend that consumers of kava should consider the following cautions:

- Kava should not be used by anyone who has liver problems, is taking any drug product with known adverse effects on the liver, or is a regular consumer of alcohol.
- Since the reports so far are associated with chronic use, kava should not be taken on a daily basis for more than the German Commission E's recommendation of three months.
- Discontinue use if symptoms of jaundice (e.g., dark urine, yellowing of the eyes) occur.
- Do not exceed the recommended maximums of 125 mg kavalactones per tablet or capsule, 3 g of dried rhizome per tea bag, and 250 mg kavalactones total per day for all forms.
- Kava should not be taken with alcohol or other sedatives because they potentiate each other (that is, they increase each other's potency). You should never drive after using kava in higher doses. There have already been a few arrests for erratic driving under the influence.
- Because high doses can cause intoxication, there is concern that kava could become an herb of abuse. There have been media reports of young people trying to get high by taking products that they thought contained kava. Exploiting its exotic appeal, people

distributed bottles of a product called "fX" and promoted it as kava at a 1996 Los Angeles New Year's Eve celebration. There were hundreds of adverse reactions, widely reported in the press as "due to kava." Unfortunately, less attention was paid a few weeks later when the police report revealed that fX contained a highly toxic industrial chemical called 1,4-butanediol—and *absolutely no kava.*

In conclusion, be aware that herbs are potent medicines and should be treated with appropriate respect regarding interactions with potential toxicity, including toxicity to the liver. However, kava's margin of safety still far surpasses that of its pharmaceutical equivalents.

For information on using kava to help in quitting tranquilizers, see Chapter 9.

Kava

How it works: Calms the limbic system, the emotional center of the brain; relaxes muscles, likely through an indirect action on GABA receptors.

Positive effects: Relaxes mind, emotions, and muscles, making it useful for headaches, backaches, and other tension; reduces excessive mental chatter; increases mental focus; expands overall awareness; no habituation, tolerance, addiction, or hangover.

Cautions: Do not drive or operate heavy machinery after use. Do not mix with alcohol, as the two substances seem to potentiate each other. Do not take while using benzodiazepines.

Dosage: As a relaxant, 60–75 mg of kavalactones two to three times daily. As a bedtime sedative, 60–250 mg of kavalactones about 30 minutes before bedtime.

Valerian: Nature's Valium

Another favorite for the treatment of anxiety is valerian (*Valeriana offici-nalis*), sometimes referred to as "Nature's Valium." Derived from the dried rhizomes and roots of this tall plant, which grows on wet soil in many countries, valerian has been used for thousands of years as a folk remedy. As a natural relaxant, it is useful for several disorders, including restlessness, nervousness, insomnia, menstrual problems, and "nervous" stomach. Valerian acts on the brain's GABA receptors to produce a tranquilizing action that is similar to Valium-type drugs, but without the same side effects.

Be forewarned, though—its smell has been likened to old socks! So hold your nose, and here's how to take it. Using standardized extract (0.8 percent valeric acid), the dose is 50–100 mg, two to three times daily for relaxation. For bedtime sedation to promote sleep, take 150–300 mg about 45 minutes before bedtime.

Another word of caution: valerian can interact with alcohol and certain antihistamines, muscle relaxants, psychotropic drugs, and narcotics. Those taking any of these drugs should take valerian only under the supervision of a health-care practitioner.

For information on using valerian to help in discontinuing tranquilizers, see Chapter 9.

Valerian

How it works: Enhances GABA activity.

Positive effects: Reduces anxiety, insomnia, and tension.

Cautions: Potentiates sedative drugs, including muscle relaxants and antihistamines; can interact with alcohol.

Dosage: As a relaxant, 50–100 mg, two to three times a day. As a bedtime sedative, 150–300 mg about 45 minutes before bedtime.

The next two plants are traditional sedating herbs that you will often find in combination formulas. Like many subtle flavorings, however, they do add their own special qualities to the mix, and you might like to know something about them.

Hops: Happy Snoozing

Hops (*Humulus lupulus*) has been used for centuries as a mild sedative and sleeping aid. The herb is primarily used to calm nerves and induce sleep, usually in combination with other herbal sedatives such as passionflower, valerian, and skullcap. Its sedative action works directly on the central nervous system. The dose is around 200 mg per day but varies from formula to formula.

Passionflower: Rest Easy

The mild sedative effect of passionflower (*Passiflora incarnata*) has been well substantiated in numerous animal and human studies. The herb encourages a deep, restful, and uninterrupted sleep, with no side effects. Passionflower has been commonly used in the treatment of concentration problems in schoolchildren and as a sedative for the elderly. In high doses, passionflower has been found to be mildly hallucinogenic, though we don't recommend trying it for that. Dosage varies with the formula but is generally 100–200 mg per day of the standardized product.

RELAXING NATURALLY WITH AMINO ACIDS

GABA: Truly Chilled

We've now heard quite a bit about GABA, the main inhibitory or calming amino acid and neurotransmitter. GABA also acts as a significant mood modulator by regulating the neurotransmitters noradrenaline, dopamine, and serotonin. GABA helps to shift a tense, worried state to relaxation, and a blue mood to a happy one. When your levels of GABA are low, you feel anxious, tense, depressed, and have trouble sleeping. When your levels increase, your breathing and heart rate slow and your muscles relax, making it a welcome addition to any chill-out program.

While you can enhance GABA activity with herbs, as we've seen, you

GABA

How it works: Acts directly on the brain as a calming, mood-enhancing neuro-transmitter.

Positive effects: Reduces anxiety, insomnia, and tension.

Cautions: Can cause nausea and vomiting at high doses.

Dosage: 250–500 mg twice daily after meals, and, if needed, again at bedtime.

can also take GABA directly in powder or pill form—100–500 mg two to three times daily, generally mid-morning, mid-afternoon, and, if needed, at bedtime. A review article on GABA by two psychiatrists at the University of British Columbia in Vancouver makes it clear that it is able to move easily from the bloodstream into the brain. In technical terms, inability to cross the blood-brain barrier is often an obstacle to a product's effectiveness. So you can be sure that the GABA you ingest will actually get to its target, the brain.

Taurine: Calming Influence

Taurine is an amino acid that plays a major role in the brain as an "in-hibitory" neurotransmitter. Similar in structure and function to GABA, tau-rine provides a similar antianxiety effect that helps to calm or stabilize an excited brain. Taurine has many other uses as well, including treating mi-graine, insomnia, agitation, restlessness, irritability, alcoholism, obsessions, depression, and even hypomania/mania—the "high" phase of bipolar disor-der or manic depression. People have also reported getting a pleasant high from taking one or two capsules!

By inhibiting the release of adrenaline, taurine also protects us from anxiety and other adverse effects of stress. It even helps control high blood pressure. You may have noticed it as an ingredient in some of the energiz-ing, high-caffeine soft drinks, to soften any overstimulation.

Taurine

How it works: Enhances GABA activity.

Positive effects: Reduces anxiety, irritability, insomnia, migraine, alcoholism, obsessions, and depression.

Cautions: None reported.

Dosage: 250–500 mg twice daily, between meals.

Vegetarians can be at risk for taurine deficiency since taurine is found in animal and fish protein, especially organ meats. A nonessential amino acid, taurine can be manufactured by the body in the liver and brain from the amino acids L-cysteine and L-methionine, plus the cofactor vitamin B_6. When there are insufficiencies, though, you are best to supplement directly with taurine. The recommended dose is 100–500 mg twice daily, and higher as needed, between meals for best absorption.

ACTION PLAN FOR NATURAL RELAXATION

There would be no point in taking any of these herbs or amino acids if you continue to eat a junk-food diet that is high in caffeine, alcohol, and sugar. You must, of course, begin with a solid base, as discussed in "Natural High Basics" in Chapter 3.

B vitamins are required for the smooth running of the nervous system and the production of adrenal or stress hormones. And certain minerals have a relaxing effect on the body and emotions. However, during stress, B vitamins and the minerals calcium, magnesium, and potassium all are depleted, leading to further anxiety. So make sure that you are taking enough of the following, especially under stressful conditions: vitamins B_1, B_3, B_6,

B_{12}, folic acid, calcium, magnesium, phosphorus, and omega-3 fatty acids, such as fish or flaxseed oil.

In other words, balance your body and provide it with the fuel it needs so that any new mood-enhancing additions will be able to do their jobs.

Getting and staying relaxed may involve making some changes. See Part Three for ways to alter your lifestyle. Changing your chemistry is just as vital, and here's how you can do it.

Balance Your Blood Sugar: An Even Keel

There are three golden rules for keeping your blood-sugar levels even:

1. Avoid, or at least considerably reduce, all sugar and stimulants (see Chapter 5 for natural alternatives).
2. Eat regularly and eat low-GI foods to keep your blood-sugar levels even.
3. Take supplements of the "energy nutrients," primarily B vitamins and vitamin C, which help to turn your food efficiently into energy.

All of this was explained in Chapter 3. If you are very stressed, or suspect you have a blood-sugar problem, you will also benefit by adding a morning dose of 200 mcg of chromium, a mineral that helps insulin to keep your blood-sugar levels stable.

Mobilize GABA: The Big Chill Out

The following herbs and amino acids help to calm the stress response and act as natural relaxants. The ideal daily doses of all of them are less when combined than when the substance is taken alone. These are all suggested ranges, since responses will vary based on your unique chemistry. Test your dose carefully, and increase as needed. Then, add in one new item at a time, and observe your response.

Since herbs are extracts, the dose will vary based on the percent of the marker in the standardized extract (see page 63). The kava dosage given here relates to the actual amount of kavalactones in the product, be it powder, capsules, or tincture.

74

Natural Relaxants	Daily Dose
Kava	60–250 mg (60–75 mg, two to three times daily; 120–150 mg, generally 1–2 capsules, at bedtime)
Valerian	50–300 mg (50–100 mg twice daily; 150–300 mg at bedtime)
Hops	100–200 mg, 2–3 times daily
Passionflower	100–200 mg, 2–3 times daily
GABA	100–500 mg, one to three times daily, between meals
Taurine	100–500 mg, one to two times daily, between meals

If not marked for between meals, products can be taken any time, with or without meals.

So, to sum up, you should take the following to chill out:

- A good all-around multivitamin supplying optimal amounts of B vitamins, vitamin C, with an optional 200 mcg of chromium.
- A "chill-out" formula providing kava, valerian, hops, passionflower, GABA, and taurine, as needed.
- For a good night's sleep, take 150–300 mg of valerian and 120–150 mg of kava about 45 minutes before bedtime, plus 200 mg of 5-HTP (see page 125). We recommend starting one new product at a time, observing your response, then adding in a new one as needed.

For a full natural chill-out program, see Top Tips in Part Four.

5

Energizers

The Exhaustion Epidemic

Let's visit childhood once more. Remember bounding out of bed in the morning, eager to meet the new day? There were playmates to visit, games to play, trees to climb, and little place for boredom or exhaustion. Look at the kids around you—there is an abiding energy and an enthusiasm that keep them going. Even in the evening, while you might be collapsing, their squirming little bodies want "just five more minutes" or "one more story" before succumbing to sleep.

Most of us would pay a high price to feel such energy. We get more done, and have more fun doing it, when we're feeling alive and alert. But somehow, as adults, most of us have outgrown this early exuberance, and we can't always summon the energy we want. We may rely instead on the use of artificial energizers.

To a large extent, the roots of our dependency on stimulants can be traced back to the Industrial Revolution, which demanded brutally long hours from workers. To meet the grueling demands of industry, workers were fueled with tea, coffee, and tobacco to stimulate them to work faster and more efficiently. Soon sugar entered the mix, to sweeten the tea and coffee, followed later by the introduction of chocolate. Ever-increasing consumption of these stimulants continued into the twentieth century, rapidly becoming part of the daily ritual of millions of people throughout Europe. And this trend continues to grow in the new millennium.

These "workers friends" aren't the only stimulants around, of course. Amphetamines, cocaine, and even alcohol—both a stimulant and a relaxant—fall into this category, too. All of these affect the emotional center of the brain—the limbic system—to produce the cherished experience of pleasure. Issues of illegality or serious health consequences aside, these popular stimulants will simply compound our load of exhaustion.

We'll be looking at the wellspring of that exhaustion and the substances that offer a quick-fix solution—which ultimately becomes part of the problem. And we'll see how it's possible to get back our energy by using ancient herbs and natural nutrients.

Our own technological revolution has spawned a world that never sleeps. Markets are open twenty-four hours; television and the Internet call to us twenty-four hours a day, seven days a week. Many of us are trying to keep impossible schedules to meet work and family responsibilities. When we shave an hour off our sleep, we feel we've gained some small advantage.

This all has a cumulative effect. You struggle to find time with your kids, friends, and colleagues, not to mention your partner. You start off less alert than you'd like, begin to feel drowsy as the day wears on, and doze off if you sit down to read or watch TV in the evening. When you finally find yourself together with your partner at bedtime, neither of you has any energy left to do anything about it!

Too often today, we rely on chemical "helpers" to keep us going: the frequent coffee breaks, the doughnut to satisfy our hunger when we have no time to eat, the cigarette to calm our nerves. You will soon see why we use stimulants, how the common stimulants affect us, how we become dependent on them, and how to replace them with healthier, more effective alternatives.

To get an idea of how depleted your energy might be and how dependent you are on stimulants, check yourself out on the Energy Check questionnaire on page 14 if you have not already done so.

An Addicted Society

Stimulant-seeking behavior carried to the extreme becomes addiction. In the United States alone, there are 6 million people addicted to cocaine, 25 million people addicted to nicotine, and 14.9 million people who abuse other substances. Of concern, too, are the large numbers of school-age children and college students who are experimenting with these substances. There are also about 54 million people who are at least 20 percent overweight—food addicts—and 448,000 compulsive gamblers.

WHAT'S UP WITH STIMULANTS?

If you give in to your cravings for stimulants, it does not necessarily mean you are weak or "bad," but simply that your chemistry is controlling you. You need the right fuel—foods, vitamins, and other micronutrients—to run your body's engine. (See Chapter 3.) You also need sufficient sleep to restore body and mind and to maintain your energy level. Chronic sleep deprivation is a major source of fatigue. (See Chapter 21.)

You might even have a medical condition such as a chronic viral infection (chronic fatigue syndrome) or an imbalance in your hormones such as an underactive thyroid gland that makes you feel exhausted. Turning to stimulants to rev up your engine only further depletes your already bankrupt system.

THE ROOTS OF ADDICTION

Addiction can also have genetic roots, since we know that addiction runs in families. Programmed by your genes, you may be hard-wired for stimulant addiction. An inborn deficiency in the number of dopamine receptors can lead to feelings of depression, low self-esteem, low energy, irritability, and lack of motivation. Termed *reward deficiency syndrome (RDS)* by researcher Kenneth Blum, the deficiency may cause sufferers to "self-medicate" in the form of drugs, alcohol, or thrill-seeking, dangerous behavior to feel energized, motivated, or happy. Alcohol and stimulant addiction can be the unfortunate result. Note, however, that RDS creates a *predisposition* only: you are not a slave to your genes. There are ways to deal with the problem nutritionally, as you will learn.

MY PARENTS MADE ME DO IT

We can also learn addictive behavior from our families as we're growing up. Joan's parents, for example, would give her chocolate as a treat or reward on special occasions. Since it reminds her of the simple pleasures of childhood, Joan still comforts herself with hot chocolate or a candy bar binge when times get rough. Many children are raised on sugared cereals and soft drinks full of caffeine and sugar, leaving them hooked. Jerry's experience is another case in point: his teenage friends smoked cigarettes, so he joined them to fit in and look cool. Now, at age forty, he is an addicted smoker.

SUMMARY

We are living unnatural lifestyles that lead to excessive stress and use of stimulants. The neurotransmitter dopamine, from which we make adrenaline and noradrenaline, is released when we are stressed or use stimulants. Motivating and pleasurable, stimulants generate energy by mobilizing glucose. As a result, stimulants make us more alert, energized, cheerful, or even high. These include sugar, chocolate, tea, coffee, cigarettes, caffeinated drinks, amphetamines, and cocaine. Downregulation quickly steps in to stop the fun. As a result, we need more and more of the stimulant to feel good and to maintain our energy levels. This leads to a vicious cycle of stimulant dependence and fatigue. Fatigue (and resultant stimulant cravings) can have many sources, including poor sleep and diet, chronic infection, and hormone imbalances. Since the stress hormones adrenaline and cortisol lead to release of dopamine, we can become addicted to our own feel-good hormones, so we create more stress to keep the cycle going.

In the next section, we will look at the common substances that we use for stimulation and what they actually do to us.

Handle with Care: Popular Stimulants

Stimulants have been around the block a few times. Since prehistory, people have used a variety of substances to energize, motivate, and inspire. Native North Americans smoked tobacco, the natives of the Andes chewed coca leaves, and Indians and Chinese drank tea. And then there are our Western offerings: sugar, tea, coffee, cigarettes, and stimulant drugs. Even some medications for the relief of headaches, such as Anacin, contain caffeine. Other caffeine tablets, such as Dexatrine, are sold outright as stimulants. In this section we will explore the effects of these substances, as well as their caffeine-containing cousins: chocolate, guarana, maté, and kola nut. We'll also look at ephedra (*ma huang*) and yohimbe.

They may be popular, but stimulants are also problematic. All stimulants work by mimicking or triggering the release of the three primary neurotransmitters: dopamine, adrenaline, and noradrenaline. That's what makes you feel motivated and high. We learned earlier how downregulation in the brain eventually puts a stop to the fun of getting high. The exact same thing happens with stimulants: overstimulation leads to downregulation, causing the receptor sites to shut down. You keep needing more of the product for the same effect. But how much is too much? And are there some stimulants we can take safely in moderation?

While a substance can make us feel good in the moment, in the long term it can actually be harmful. In one short-term experiment, coffee was shown to heighten alertness (as if we didn't know!), but the researchers weren't looking at the memory impairment or increased blood pressure in habitual coffee drinkers. Also, researchers are not always without bias and may interpret results to fit their preconceptions or desired outcome.

We'll deal with these issues as we discuss each substance in detail. But for now, we can say that some stimulants are never recommended, while others can be acceptable in moderation, depending on the situation.

POPULAR STIMULANTS

Sugar: Toxic Treat

Sugar is a fairly recent entry into the stimulant game. Of course, it's always been available in natural sources such as fruit, with its slow-releasing fructose, balanced by the fiber content. Refined sugar, however, only came in with the Industrial Revolution. Today, we can hardly picture a celebration without sweet treats—birthday and wedding cakes, Halloween candy, and Christmas candy canes. Every religion and culture have their celebratory sweets.

How can such a delicious and seemingly harmless treat be so damaging? Stripped of its fiber and nutrients, highly refined sugar is rapidly absorbed and broken down into molecules of glucose that quickly reach the brain to produce feelings of "comfort" or "energy." Sugar binging looks a lot like any other addiction—tolerance develops, and you need more to get the same effect. How serious is that?

DOWNSIDE OF SUGAR   Excess sugar is bad for you. While sugar is valuable fuel for our cells, it can be toxic when consumed in excess, often causing damage to the arteries, kidneys, eyes, and nerves. The body tries to get it out of the blood and into storage as quickly as possible, but this can then cause a "rebound" low blood-sugar effect with its own set of problems. Some people feel stimulated immediately after eating it, then become cranky and finally go into a low blood-sugar slump.

Caffeine: Brewing Up Trouble

Found in more than one hundred plants throughout the world, caffeine is consumed primarily in beverages. A half-dozen caffeine-containing plants are more widely used than all other herbal materials combined!

More than a thousand years ago, Muslims used coffee for religious rituals. Finally reaching Europe in the seventeenth century, it was seen by the authorities as a dangerous drug. Nonetheless, coffeehouses spread, as did dependence on this new drug. The rest is history. Together with tea, it comprises 97 percent of worldwide caffeine consumption. Some parts of the world use other forms of caffeine—guarana, maté, and kola nut—which are now becoming more popular in the West.

Caffeine was first isolated from coffee in 1821. The effects of coffee are more potent than those of caffeine alone, since it contains two other stimulants—theophylline and theobromine. These weaker versions of caffeine are also found in decaffeinated coffee. All three are xanthines, alkaloid compounds that occur in both plants and animals.

The main reason we drink caffeine is that it boosts mood and energy. It does this by blocking the receptors for a brain chemical called *adenosine*, whose function is to stop dopamine release. With less adenosine activity, then, you increase dopamine and adrenaline. You feel alert, motivated, and stimulated, though some people will feel uncomfortable and jittery. Caffeine reaches its peak concentration in 30–60 minutes, after which it is inactivated by the liver, with only half its peak level left after 4–6 hours.

So where's the danger? Caffeine is addictive. Research shows that consuming as little as 100 mg a day can lead to withdrawal symptoms when you stop, including headache, fatigue, difficulty concentrating, and drowsiness. It's worth knowing that, while a small cup of instant coffee may contain less than 100 mg of caffeine, a large cup of "designer" coffee can contain as much as 500 mg—five times the "addictive" dose. Even more chemicals are used in manufacturing decaffeinated coffee, and, in the end, it still contains traces of caffeine—about 0.5 mg per 8-ounce cup.

DOWNSIDE OF CAFFEINE

- Overstimulated central nervous system, leading to increased risk of heart attacks, irritability, insomnia, and rapid and irregular heartbeats.
- Elevated blood pressure (hypertension).
- Elevated blood-sugar and cholesterol levels.
- Heartburn and other gastrointestinal problems.
- Fibrocystic breast disease.
- Diuresis (excessive urination), which can lead to dehydration.
- Increased risk of birth defects if used during pregnancy.
- Contains tars, phenols, and other carcinogens, as well as traces of pesticides and toxic chemicals used in the growing and extraction processes.

At best, we can say that coffee has minor short-term mental and emotional benefits but that these are not sustained. A study published in the *American Journal of Psychiatry* observed 1,500 psychology students divided into four categories depending on their coffee intake: abstainers; low consumers (1 cup or equivalent a day); moderate (1–5 cups a day); and high (5 cups or more a day). On psychological testing, the moderate and high consumers had higher levels of anxiety and depression than the abstainers, and the high consumers had higher incidence of stress-related medical problems coupled with lower academic performance.

The bottom line? Drink coffee in moderation, if at all.

Tea: Not So Refreshing

Tea (*Camellia sinensis*) has been a favorite stimulant in many countries for centuries. Black tea is prepared by the initial slow drying of the fresh leaves, which allows them to begin to ferment, while for green tea, the leaves are dried quickly. Both contain caffeine.

The drinking of tea began in ancient Asia, and by the seventeenth century, the beverage had been adopted as Britain's standard refresher. By the early nineteenth century, as we've seen, tea had become a highly sought-after stimulant in the newly industrializing society, providing energy to goad the workers into faster production. And as tea required lots of sugar to enhance its bitter taste, the economy got another boost from sugar sales.

Tea continues to be a significant pick-me-up and social ritual in Britain, where tea consumption is four times that of coffee. In the United States, the figures are reversed. You can guess why by recalling the historic Boston Tea Party, which preceded the American Revolution. Rather than pay a tea tax to their oppressors across the sea, the colonists dumped boxes of imported tea from British trade ships into the harbor—and haven't had much taste for it since.

Tea's stimulating effects come from the same compounds as in coffee—caffeine, theobromine, and theophylline. Because of different methods of preparation and the many varieties of the cultivated plant, the average caffeine content of tea ranges widely from about 1 percent to more than 4 percent. The downsides of drinking tea are mentioned below. However, green tea does have some redeeming features (see page 107).

DOWNSIDE OF TEA A strong cup of tea contains as much caffeine as a weak cup of coffee—with all the attendant risks mentioned on page 82. Also, the tannin content of tea interferes with the absorption of minerals.

The Cola Generation

Cola drinks contain about one-quarter to one-half of the caffeine found in a weak cup of coffee. One cola drink even contained small amounts of coca (cocaine) in its original formula, hence the name, Coca-Cola. We also have non-cola caffeinated soft drinks such as Mountain Dew. Today's drinks generally contain sugar and colorings, which are also stimulants. Maybe worse, diet drinks contain the artificial sweetener aspartame (Nutrasweet), which can be toxically overstimulating to the brain. We have seen people who thought they were "going crazy" with jitters, insomnia, and disordered thinking magically recover when they stopped drinking diet sodas. Ironically, although touted as a diet product, these drinks can actually cause weight gain. See http://www.dorway.com/blayenn.html for scientific information on aspartame.

More recently, new soft drinks have been introduced that push up the levels of caffeine they contain, boosting both their kick and addictiveness. Shades of the tobacco industry! With names such as Jolt or Red Bull, their caffeine content can equal or even surpass that of a cup of coffee. Children and young people are drinking large amounts of caffeinated soft drinks, especially relative to their weight, exposing their developing brains and bodies to a hazardous substance. Never mind illicit drugs—junk food and caffeinated drinks can lead to serious health problems and addictions in children.

DOWNSIDE OF COLAS
- Contain caffeine—with all the attendant risks.
- Sugar and coloring are added stimulants; aspartame in diet colas can toxically overstimulate the brain.
- Newer cola drinks aimed at young people have even higher levels of caffeine.

Caffeine Buzzometer
(Caffeine Levels of Common Products)

PRODUCT	CAFFEINE CONTENT *(per serving)*
Coca-Cola Classic 350 ml (12 fl oz)	45 mg
Diet Coke 350 ml (12 fl oz)	45 mg
Red Bull 250 ml (8.3 fl oz)	80 mg
Hot cocoa 150 ml (5 fl oz)	10 mg
Coffee, instant 150 ml (5 fl oz)	40–105 mg
Espresso, cappuccino, or latte (single)	30–50 mg
Coffee, filter 150 ml (5 fl oz)	110–150 mg
Coffee, Starbucks grande	500 mg
Coffee, decaffeinated 150 ml (5 fl oz)	0.3 mg
Tea 150 ml (5 fl oz)	20–100 mg
Green tea 150 ml (5 fl oz)	15–30 mg
Chocolate cake (1 slice)	20–30 mg
Bittersweet chocolate (1 oz)	5–35 mg
Excedrin (2 tablets)	130 mg
NoDoz (2 capsules)	200 mg
Dexatrim (1 500-mg capsule)	80 mg

Death by Chocolate?

Chocolate's major active ingredient is cocoa, a significant source of the stimulant theobromine. Research by British psychologist, Dr. David Benton at the University of Wales in Swansea, found chocolate to be an excellent mood elevator. When he played sad music to a group of students, their moods sank. He then offered them the choice of milk chocolate or carob, a natural chocolate substitute that is similar in taste. Without their knowing which product they were eating, the participants found that the chocolate raised their moods, while the carob didn't. Moreover, as their moods fell, their cravings for chocolate increased.

In addition to theobromine—which is also found in tea and coffee—chocolate also contains the mood-enhancing stimulant phenethylamine. Both theobromine and phenethylamine stimulate dopamine production. Even experimental alcohol-loving rats, when given the choice, will replace some of their alcohol intake with chocolate.

A recent study of mice and rats shows that dopamine kick-starts a brain messenger chemical called DARP-32, which in turn activates hormones that make females more interested in sex. Without even knowing about DARP-32, generations of lonely, frustrated men and women have binged on chocolate, with sometimes surprising results. Valentine's Day chocolates say it all.

The bad news? Too much chocolate, especially the highly sweetened kind, causes all the problems of going overboard on sugar, including weight gain. Chocolate is often high in fats, too. The addictive nature of chocolate suggests the development of tolerance, and "just one piece of chocolate" becomes, instead, "just one *more*." In addition, like coffee, cocoa beans are often grown in countries where pesticide use is unregulated, exposing the consumer to cancer-causing compounds.

If you are going to eat chocolate, eat the pure, dark, preferably organic type, not cheap bars full of fat and sugar. But, as with any stimulant, if you eat chocolate every day, or find yourself craving it, you've gone too far. Keep chocolate as a special treat, not a daily ritual.

DOWNSIDE OF CHOCOLATE
- Contains caffeine—with all the attendant risks.
- Often high in sugar and fats, leading to weight gain.
- May be treated with carcinogenic pesticides in country of origin.

Guarana, Maté, Kola Nut: Caffeine by Any Other Name
The name *guarana* conjures up exotic images of tribal people in the Amazonian rain forests, living in harmony with nature. And if it's "natural," it must be good for you. Right? Well, not exactly. The seeds and leaves of the guarana plant, a climbing shrub native to Brazil and Uruguay, are high in caffeine.

Once a traditional social drink, appetite suppressant, and aphrodisiac, guarana is used extensively in South America today in soft drinks. Because it contains saponins—compounds found in ginseng—native preparations may possess tonic or balancing properties. They are less irritating to the gastrointestinal tract than say, coffee, and also have a mild and long-lasting effect. This is probably due to the presence of fats and oils in the seeds, which prolong absorption. On the other hand, most commercially prepared products are absorbed and used up in the body as quickly as a cup of coffee. Once again, the closer we stick to the natural form of a product, the healthier it is for us.

A dried paste made chiefly from the crushed seed of guarana has a relatively high caffeine content, ranging from 2.5 to 5 percent, and averaging about 3.5 percent. To determine how much caffeine is in any product, you must do your math: multiply the total weight of the capsule or powder by the percentage of caffeine or guarana to get the number of milligrams of caffeine per dose.

The conclusion regarding its use? Like tea or coffee, guarana can be overstimulating and have the same ill effects. In a dilute, milder form, guarana can be used as an occasional pick-me-up for those whose adrenal status is healthy—that is, not suffering from stress or burnout.

Another traditional South American stimulant is the jungle tea *maté* (pronounced "ma-*tay*"). The dried leaves of this low-growing bush are brewed into a hot drink. Besides low concentrations of caffeine, maté contains theophylline (0.05 percent), theobromine (0.1 to 2 percent), tannins, vitamins, and minerals. At 15–25 mg of caffeine per cup, as in green tea, maté is used for enhancing alertness and concentration. It can be useful on occasion, certainly better than most stimulants mentioned here. As with any stimulant, excessive use can tax the adrenal glands.

Kola nut is used as an aphrodisiac, probably working the same way as chocolate. The nut (*Cola nitida*) is a seed kernel related to the cacao tree, and is native to the rain forests of West Africa. It is also cultivated in the West Indies and other tropical areas. Containing up to 3 percent caffeine, its stimulant properties were originally derived from chewing on the seeds. Kola nut is now available as tea made of ground seeds. Kola nut was the "cola" part of coke, which, as we mentioned earlier, also originally contained coca extract. Cola drinks now get their kick from synthesized or extracted caffeine plus sugar.

Downsides of Guarana, Maté, and Kola Nut

- All contain caffeine—with all the attendant risks.
- Guarana and maté can only be used by those with healthy adrenal status—not the seriously stressed.

Ephedra (Ma Huang): Life in the Fast Lane

Though a traditional remedy with a long history of medical use, ephedra has recently become a controversial herb—within both the natural products industry and government regulatory agencies—because of its misuse. Called *ma huang (Ephedra sinica)*, this ancient Chinese remedy triggers the release of adrenaline, the hormone that mediates the stress response. Since the stress response also causes an initial surge in energy, as well as suppression of appetite, ephedra is often used for both quick energy and weight loss. One study found that it worked better than Redux, a weight loss drug that was later withdrawn from the market because of its toxic effects. A 1996 study found that a combination of 30 mg of ephedra, 100 mg of caffeine, and 300 mg of aspirin promoted fat-burning. Ephedra is also used as a decongestant, most commonly as ephedrine, a more potent and longer-lasting synthetic version of ephedra.

Ephedra is also used by some for recreation. Advertised as "herbal Ecstasy," ephedra actually has little in common with the entheogen Ecstasy, or MDMA (see Chapter 8). Rather, what's marketed as herbal Ecstasy is generally a combination of ephedra and caffeine—both in high doses—which causes a "rush" that is stimulating and energizing. The high-dose combination can be dangerous, however, producing a rapid heart rate and a rise in blood pressure with accompanying headache, dizziness, and, on rare occasions, even death.

Having the right information will help you choose whether or not to use ephedra. Doses of ephedra should not exceed 8 mg per dose or 24 mg per day. If used at all, ephedra should be taken for short periods of time—days, not weeks or months. Athletes often use ephedra as a stimulant, and while it may increase exercise tolerance, the risk of heart problems is certainly not worth it. We have already seen young athletes, perhaps with undiagnosed preexisting heart problems, have a sudden heart arrhythmia, some fatal, in association with taking ephedra-containing supplements. Nor is it advised for people with diabetes, heart conditions, or those who are energy depleted, recovering from any illness, suffering from a weak constitution, or just hypersensitive to it.

DOWNSIDE OF EPHEDRA Below are some of the negative side effects associated with ephedra at higher than the recommended doses:

- Headache, tremor, insomnia, and anxiety.
- Rapid heart rate, irregular heart rhythm, and a rise in blood pressure.
- Increased risk of heart attack, seizure, or stroke in susceptible individuals.
- Reversible toxic psychosis from overstimulation of the brain.
- A weakened heart, adrenals, and other organs in the long term.

CONTRAINDICATIONS Ephedra should not be taken by children, pregnant or breast-feeding women, or people with diabetes, high blood pressure, heart problems, thyroid problems, or psychiatric disorders. Consult with a health-care practitioner prior to use if you have difficulty urinating, prostate enlargement, or glaucoma, or are using any prescription drug. It should not be taken in combination with the so-called "MAOI" antidepressant drugs (see Chapter 6), or cold medication containing ephedrine pseudo-ephedrine, or phenylpropanolamine. Discontinue if sleepiness, dizziness, loss of appetite, or nausea occurs.

The natural products industry has taken action to educate the public and to provide quality, safe products. Such organizations include the Ephedra Committee of the American Herbal Products Association and the American Botanical Council. Many countries restrict the use of ephedra. The Canadian health agency recently recalled all ephedra products that make weight-loss or stimulant claims, that are manufactured in combination with stimulants (e.g., caffeine and caffeine-containing herbs), or that exceed the federal dosage levels (i.e., more than 8 mg of ephedrine per dose, 25 mg per day, and recommended for longer than a seven-day period). Ephedra/ephedrine products that are marketed as traditional medicines or are sold as nasal decongestants continue to be available, provided that they comply with the federal dosage levels and do not contain caffeine.

In the U.K., ephedra is available only by prescription by registered herbalists and pharmacists. In the United States, ephedra is currently available without prescription. Due to adverse events reports, the F.D.A. has proposed dosage limits and is considering other restrictions including an outright ban of the herb. In the summer of 2001, the *New England Journal of Medicine* released a study of the effects of ephedra six months early because the *Journal* considered the findings sufficiently negative and important.

Yohimbe: The Sexy Herb

The traditional African herb yohimbe is as controversial a stimulant as ephedra. In its extracted alkaloid form, yohimbine, it is used not only as a mood enhancer and weight-loss product but also as a male aphrodisiac. In fact, yohimbine hydrochloride in 5.4-mg tablets is prescribed by doctors to treat impotence.

Yohimbe enhances the stimulant neurotransmitters, dopamine and noradrenaline. As with other stimulants, it affects people differently. For some, there is a pleasant enhancement of the senses, an increase in empathy and communication, and enhanced sexual arousal. Men can have longer-lasting erections and powerful ejaculations. But others feel uncomfortably stimulated, with rapid heart rate, headache, anxiety, and insomnia. Yohimbe can also cause a dangerous rise in blood pressure.

The bottom line? Yohimbe appears safe for occasional use, with the proper precautions. It should not be taken by those with any cardiovascular condition.

DOWNSIDE OF YOHIMBE In susceptible individuals, it can cause uncomfortable overstimulation—rapid heart rate, headache, anxiety, insomnia, and a dangerous rise in blood pressure. Avoid liver, cheeses, red wine, nasal decongestants, and diet aids.

CONTRAINDICATIONS Yohimbe should not be taken by people suffering from any cardiovascular condition, diabetes, or heart, liver, or kidney disease.

DEFINITE NO'S: FROM SMOKING TO SPEED

The Tobacco High

Together with caffeine and alcohol, nicotine is one of the three most widely used psychoactive drugs in our society. With no redeeming value, "smoking will continue as the leading cause of preventable, premature mortality for many years to come," according to the U.S. Surgeon General. In 1997, smoking killed 435,000 people in the United States alone.

Nicotine, the primary stimulant in cigarettes, has a significant effect, even in small doses. In fact, nicotine is such a powerful toxin that one cigar contains enough to kill several people (and not just from the smell)!

If you have ever smoked, can you recall the sensation of your first cigarette? It probably tasted terrible, burned your mouth and lungs (if you even inhaled), and made you feel nauseated and dizzy. Those are some of its toxic effects in action. After a few more smokes, your body no longer rebels. In fact, you rather like it. In short—you're hooked.

Nicotine has a complex series of actions, both stimulating and relaxing. It is more addictive than heroin—and is often the hardest addiction to break. Nicotine stimulates the adrenals to release adrenaline, raising blood pressure and heart rate, and increases gastrointestinal activity. Nicotine also acts as a muscle relaxant.

In the brain, nicotine activates the release of dopamine, exhibiting a stimulant effect similar to that of caffeine. It also has a short-term antidepressant effect, though this is most often followed by a rebound depression. In larger amounts, nicotine acts as a sedative, probably because of its effect on serotonin. People trying to kick the tobacco habit describe the accompanying tension and irritability as "feeling like you want to jump out of your skin." They also often experience low blood-sugar problems, which leads them to overeat and gain weight.

For details on how to stop smoking, see Chapter 9.

Cocaine: Ups and Downs

Cocaine is probably the best-known—and most powerful—illegal stimulant. The active ingredient of the coca plant, cocaine was first isolated in the West around 1860. The father of psychoanalysis, Sigmund Freud, personally experimented with the refined powdered drug and described cocaine as "magical." While the coca leaf typically contains between 0.1 and 0.9 percent cocaine, concentrated coca paste contains up to 60 to 80 percent pure cocaine. The drug works by blocking the reabsorption of dopamine, which leaves more in the synapse to interact with the receptors.

The coca leaf, as found in nature, is safely used by field laborers in the Andes to maintain energy. The concentrated drug, however, leads to an intense "rush," with enhanced mood, sensory awareness, self-confidence, and sexual interest. Unfortunately, this is generally followed by a crash into anxiety, depression, irritability, and exhaustion. If the vicious cycle of addiction ensues, there is an intense craving for the next hit, and users follow a downhill course of deteriorating physical and mental health—often emerging as severe depression, agitation, and even paranoia.

Amphetamines: Mother's Little Uppers

Popularly known as "speed," amphetamines have been used for years by long-distance truck drivers, students cramming for finals, and harried housewives needing a lift. Like cocaine, amphetamine blocks neurons' reabsorption of the neurotransmitters noradrenaline and dopamine, but it also triggers their release, doubling its potency.

Amphetamines were discovered in the 1930s and commonly prescribed by the 1960s. In contrast with little "happy pills," these were stimulating ones that allowed users to do more, focus better, and feel more energized—until the pill wore off and they needed another fix. These drugs were later used as diet pills and as a treatment for attention deficit disorder (ADD). We have seen how women with food cravings, weight problems, depression, and even ADD were given the perfect happy pill for their condition—until the prescription ran out.

Doctors thought they were helping these women but actually turned them into addicts. Legislation then became more rigorous, and in the 1980s, the number of these prescriptions fell. The 1990s brought a resurgence, with the mushrooming of medical diet centers, dispensing stimulants such as Fen-Phen and Redux, later found to be dangerous and subsequently removed from the market.

Chronic stimulant users find it difficult to relax, and so they use relaxants such as alcohol, sleeping pills, tranquilizers, and marijuana to bring them down. This addictive cycle impairs performance, promotes stress, and depletes energy.

Amphetamines such as dexedrine and its relative, Ritalin, continue to be prescribed for children with ADD. While stimulants may work for ADD in the short term, we have found that we can prescribe natural nutrients (including amino acids) that not only work just as well in many cases but also provide the missing elements, rather than just covering the symptoms. Children show marked improvements in both behavior and grades after strategic foods such as sugar (from breakfast cereals to doughnuts) and caffeine (in the form of cola drinks) are removed from their diet. A good resource on the subject is Marcia Zimmerman's *The ADD Nutrition Solution* (www.thenutritionsolution.com).

If you are well nourished and your chemistry is well balanced, there is simply no need—or, generally, no desire—to use any of these stimulants. Then, on the odd occasion when you really need an extra lift, a small amount will have a big effect. However, in the next section, we introduce natural alternatives without the costly downsides.

Natural Energizers: A Better Boost

So now we know what to actively avoid on the stimulant front, or just handle with care. But what about mornings, always a bad time for some of us, or in those moments when we're really drained? The good news is that there are a number of substances that can give us a boost without compromising our health.

These safe and natural supplements don't deplete our reserves. Instead they help us to:

- Sustain our energy.
- Raise our spirits.
- Optimize our performance.
- Overcome our cravings to addictive stimulants.

They're nonaddictive, and the same dose will give you the same response, consistently.

ADAPTOGENS: SUPPORT YOUR ADRENALS

Since the adrenal glands are the foundation of natural energy and stimulation, we will start by looking at your level of adrenal health. Check your score on the Stress questionnaire on page 13. If your score is above 40, chances are your adrenal glands are depleted. Use the recommendations in the following section to help to restore their function. Remember, if you are stressed out, don't use stimulants, which can cause further burnout.

While Western medicine tends to ignore adrenal function unless it is either extremely low or high, traditional Chinese medicine (TCM) has subtle ways of diagnosing and treating adrenal overuse and burnout. It relies on the principles of balancing the opposites in the mind, body, and spirit. The goal is to restore the natural flow of energy using specific herbs called *adaptogens*. These herbs help the body adapt to a range of stresses, such as heat, cold, exertion, trauma, sleep deprivation, toxic exposure, radiation, infection, and psychological stress. They have few, if any, side effects, are effective for treating a wide variety of illnesses, and help return the body to homeostasis—its natural balance. By supporting and rebuilding the system in this way, adaptogens promote feelings of increased energy and well-being, with no tolerance, downregulation, or addiction.

Several groups of products help restore and enhance energy. These are the "adaptogenic" herbs, amino acids, and vitamins.

Adaptogenic herbs include ginseng (Siberian, Asian, or American), ashwaganda, licorice, reishi mushroom, and rhodiola. The stimulating amino acids include phenylalanine and tyrosine, while vitamins include pantothenic acid (vitamin B_5) and vitamin C, needed to make adrenaline and cortisol. Finally, three other substances—green tea, coenzyme NADH, and coenzyme Q_{10}—are also excellent additions to your anti-exhaustion arsenal.

Taking these substances won't give you the kind of instant jolt you'd expect from a cup of coffee or a cigarette, or the intensity of cocaine or amphetamines, but they deliver a consistent and more sustainable level of energy, alertness, and well-being. Once you feel this good, your desire for stimulants will fall away. See Chapter 9 for guidelines to help speed up the process of withdrawal from addictive substances.

The more stressful your lifestyle, the more nutrients you need. To complete your program, add the energizing and de-stressing exercises covered in Part Three.

Ginseng: King of Tonics

In continuous use in China for more than 2,000 years, ginseng, called "the king of all tonics," restores vital energy throughout the entire body, helping to overcome stress and fatigue and to recover from weakness and deficiencies. There are actually three different herbs commonly called ginseng: Siberian ginseng (*Eleutherococcus senticosus*), Asian ginseng (*Panax ginseng*), and American ginseng (*Panax quinquefolius*). The Siberian herb is not really ginseng at all, but the Russian scientists who researched it found that it functions nearly identically.

Asian ginseng is a perennial that grows in northern China, Korea, and Russia. In traditional Chinese terms, Asian ginseng is seen as more *yang*, or stimulating, than *yin*. It raises body temperature, improves digestion, strengthens the lungs, and calms the spirit. Its close relative, American ginseng, is cultivated in the United States, though largely exported to Asia. It is prized there as a *yin* herb—less heating, less stimulating, and more balanced than Asian ginseng.

The active ingredients in ginseng are called ginsenosides. There are many different ones, each having its own specific effects. Most of the modern-day research has been done on the clinical effects of single components. In 1988, a German university professor, E. Ploss, published a summary and analysis of studies on the clinical use of Asian ginseng, followed in 1990 by a review by U. Sonnenborn and Y. Proppert. All together, these articles surveyed thirty-seven experiments done between 1968 and 1990, on a total of 2,562 cases, with treatments averaging two to three months. In thirteen studies, the individuals showed an improvement in mood, and in eleven, improvement in intellectual performance. All showed a near absence of side effects.

Ginseng is available as powdered root in capsules or tablets, or as an alcohol-based tincture. The recommended dose is 100–200 mg daily of a standardized extract containing 4 to 7 percent ginsenosides.

The Russians have been far ahead of us in their recognition of Siberian ginseng, which is a valuable, less costly ginsenglike herb. In the 1940s, a Russian scientist concluded that Siberian ginseng was as good as the "real" ginsengs. Russian athletes take Siberian ginseng for months before the Olympics. Cosmonauts take it to remain alert and energetic, to help with the physical and mental stresses of life in space. It can be taken for a longer time than chemical products, since it is less stimulating.

Besides protecting the body from stress, Siberian ginseng also increases oxygenation of the cells, thereby increasing endurance and the ability to handle heavy workloads, and it improves alertness and visual-motor coordination. Siberian ginseng also tones up the body while adjusting and normalizing blood pressure and blood-sugar levels. It has the rare ability to boost both immediate and long-term energy. Research shows Siberian ginseng to be effective in improving intellectual performance and enhancing mental stamina. This makes it useful in the elderly, particularly when combined with ginkgo.

Whether you're overworked, exhausted, coping with a hangover, or involved in a taxing job such as long-distance driving, ginseng is an ideal antidote. In these cases, short-term use is all you need to get you through the emergency. It can be used safely in the long term, as well, to help you cope with the stresses of daily life.

Siberian ginseng is taken at a dose of 200–400 mg daily of standardized extract, containing greater than 1 percent eleutherosides. The dose of tincture is 5 ml twice daily of a 1:5 concentration (that is, 5 parts alcohol to 1 part ginseng).

Siberian ginseng is the safest and healthiest known stimulant, with generally no side effects. It contains no steroids or other dangerous chemical agents. It does not have the depressing qualities or addictive potential of most other pharmacological and biological stimulants, such as caffeine, amphetamines, and cocaine. It doesn't "stress" the system in stimulating it and doesn't provoke any downregulation.

As with any substance, however, allergy can occur with ginseng. Menstrual abnormalities and breast tenderness have been reported with Asian ginseng; so, for women, Siberian ginseng is often recommended instead. Overuse can cause overstimulation, including insomnia in those who are in a more advanced stage of adrenal exhaustion. Unconfirmed reports of excessive doses raising blood pressure and increasing heart rate have been largely discredited. In traditional Chinese medicine, ginseng is prescribed for pregnant women, but, as with any herb, pregnant women should use ginseng only under the care of a health-care practitioner.

According to Chinese tradition, ginseng is best used as part of a two-month restoration program. This is a time to gather and store energy, with a plan that incorporates exercise, rest, and relaxation, and avoidance of stress, drugs, and alcohol. Coupled with regular ginseng intake, this approach helps to build reserves of energy and vitality. Traditional sources recommend that you take a short break from ginseng after this renewal period. After that, it can be used as a tonic as needed. The German Commission E, a body similar to the U.S. Food and Drug Administration (FDA), concurs, recommending no more than three months at a time on any of the ginsengs, including Siberian.

Maureen's case is a good example of the appropriate use of ginseng:

> *Maureen, a forty-year-old actress, complained of being exhausted for the previous six months. She had trouble sleeping, couldn't get out of bed in the morning, and would collapse after only 15 minutes of light exercise. I prescribed Siberian ginseng (200 mg, twice daily), along with*

Siberian, Asian, and American Ginseng

How they work: Adaptogenic; support the adrenal glands.

Positive effects: Enhance the body's response to stress; decrease feelings of anxiety and stress; increase immediate energy (stimulant); restore vitality, energy, and endurance over time (tonic); increase mental and physical performance.

Cautions: None for Siberian ginseng. For Asian ginseng, possible menstrual abnormalities and breast tenderness. Overuse may cause overstimulation, including insomnia in sensitive individuals. Take a one-month break after three months of taking ginseng.

Dosage: 200–400 mg daily of Siberian ginseng; *or* 100–200 mg daily of Asian or American ginseng (standardized extract containing 4 to 7 percent ginsenosides).

licorice root and reishi mushrooms. Within four weeks, she was sleeping well and felt rested, able to get up easily in the morning. She was even able to exercise moderately for 30 minutes with no fatigue.

Ashwaganda: Indian Ginseng

An herb from India used in traditional Ayurvedic medicine, ashwaganda (*Withania somnifera*), also known as Indian ginseng, is increasingly being integrated into Western herbal practice. A versatile adaptogen, ashwaganda can enhance the immune system, boost energy, calm the stress response, and reduce levels of the stress hormone cortisol. It can also enhance memory and mental acuity due to its antioxidant effect and ability to increase acetylcholine-receptor activity. On top of all this, it's an aphrodisiac!

Ashwaganda also increases thyroid hormone levels and basal body temperature—speeding up the metabolism—in some people. In a study on animals with arthritis, ashwaganda proved better at reducing symptoms than hydrocortisone, suggesting that it has potent effects on adrenal hormone balance.

Ashwaganda

How it works: Adaptogen; stabilizes cortisol levels; acetylcholine enhancer.

Positive effects: Both energizes and calms; reduces high cortisol levels; enhances libido, memory, and cognition.

Cautions: None.

Dosage: 300 mg of a standardized extract, providing 1.5 percent of withanolides, two to three times daily.

Licorice: Balancing Act

Licorice root *(Glycyrrhiza glabra)* provides support for the adrenal glands, helping with mild adrenal insufficiency and hypoglycemia. It is also used in women for its estrogen-balancing properties. It stimulates the adrenal cortex to elevate cortisol and adrenal sex hormones by preventing their breakdown. So if you take licorice, the cortisol you make lasts longer. While we have repeatedly talked about cortisol as negative, it is essential in the short-term handling of stress. Only under chronic stress does it become a problem.

Licorice helps to raise low blood pressure, which often accompanies chronic fatigue, but this can also lead to hypertension (high blood pressure) in susceptible individuals. To avoid this side effect, the deglycyrrhinized form is used in many instances, such as in treating ulcers, but then the hormonal effect is lost.

Licorice

How it works: Prevents the breakdown of cortisol, thereby raising cortisol levels.

Positive effects: Improves adrenal function; raises low blood pressure.

Cautions: Can raise blood pressure in susceptible individuals. Not recommended for those with raised cortisol levels.

Dosage: 500 mg twice a day, morning and midday, not in the evening.

Reishi Mushroom

The glossy red or black cap of this Chinese mushroom looks unusual, especially to Western eyes. Inside are phytochemicals (plant chemicals) that make it one of the most respected tonics in herbal medicine. In Asia, especially in China and Japan, it has been revered for 5,000 years. Chinese reishi mushroom *(Ganodermum lucidum)* is often used to modify or enhance the effects of other stress-fighting herbs. With multiple benefits, it has no significant side effects.

You can use it to calm your mind, sharpen your thinking, and energize you when you feel fatigued. Reishi can even lower high blood pressure. Says herbalist Christopher Hobbs: "I often take reishi myself and have experienced immediate calming and sleep-promoting effects. I have noticed an amazing feeling in my chest with some reishi extracts, as if my heart area has 'opened up.' This unique effect, while not scientifically proven, is entirely enjoyable and often is accompanied by a feeling of immediate serenity." This certainly sounds like a natural high!

Reishi Mushroom

How it works: Adaptogen; stabilizes adrenal hormones.

Positive effects: Both calms and energizes; lowers blood pressure; sharpens mental function.

Cautions: None.

Dosage: In tincture form (20 percent), 10 ml three times a day; as tablets, 1,000 mg, in individual doses of one to three tablets three times a day.

Rhodiola (Rhodiola Rosea)
Another amazing adaptogen from the East with a long history of use is rhodiola. Growing in the Arctic regions of eastern Siberia, it is also called Arctic root. Folklore says that "those who drink rhodiola tea regularly will live more than 100 years." Chinese emperors, in search of the elixir of life, would send expeditions to Siberia to bring back this potent herb.

But it isn't all folklore. Modern science has confirmed that rhodiola has many proven benefits. Among them are its ability to improve energy, balance stress hormones, improve mood, and boost immunity. As an adaptogen, it appears to be at least as powerful as ginseng, and it protects against high levels of the stress hormone cortisol. However, rhodiola also stimulates both mental and physical performance. For this reason, it was used in the Soviet Union to improve athletic powers.

Rhodiola's effects on the brain are perhaps the most interesting. Numerous studies have shown it to improve concentration, especially in tired individuals. In one proofreading test, those taking rhodiola decreased their number of errors by 88 percent! It also helps the brain produce serotonin, which is a key "happy" neurotransmitter. In one study, 128 people suffering from depression were given 200 mg of rhodiola. Two-thirds of the patients (65 percent) had major reduction or complete disappearance of their symptoms. On top of this, rhodiola boosts immunity and has proven anticancer properties.

As with other herbs, make sure you are getting the real thing. There are many plant varieties of rhodiola, but the one that works is called *Rhodiola rosea*. While it has many active ingredients, the key components are called rosavin and salidroside. So it is best to take rhodiola supplements that are standardized and can therefore guarantee at least 2 percent rosavin and 1 percent salidroside.

Rhodiola

How it works: Adaptogen; stabilizes adrenal hormones; promotes serotonin production.

Positive effects: Improves concentration, stress resistance, physical performance, and mood; boosts immunity.

Cautions: None.

Dosage: 100 mg of standardized extract two to three times daily with meals.

STIMULATING AMINO ACIDS: LIVEN UP YOUR BRAIN

Certain amino acids are essential for brain function because they provide the building blocks (precursors) for neurotransmitters and hormones. Essential, too, are the vitamin and mineral cofactors needed to convert the amino acids into neurotransmitters (see Figure 2 on page 103). The key brain-stimulating amino acids are phenylalanine and tyrosine, which enhance all of the following: mood, energy, sexual interest, mental performance, and memory.

Since amino acids are found in high-protein foods, including meat, fish, and eggs, you might think that the way to increase your amino-acid levels would be just to eat more of these foods. However, each protein supplies a different combination of amino acids. People who have specific amino-acid deficiencies or increased needs due to prolonged stress, for instance, will require more specific supplementation.

For the best results, follow the instructions below for each of the amino acids. Since certain amino acids compete with others for transport into the brain, they are best taken separately from each other, and away from other proteins, as well. On the other hand, practicality reigns, and it's better to take them together than not at all.

Phenylalanine: Natural Caffeine

Found in meats, wheat germ, dairy products, granola, chocolate, and oatmeal, phenylalanine is an essential amino acid. It is converted by the body into tyrosine, which in turn is converted into the neurotransmitters dopamine, noradrenaline, and adrenaline. It acts like natural caffeine but without the downside.

Phenylalanine becomes depleted in cases of chronic stress and burnout, as well as by overuse of stimulant drugs such as cocaine, speed, and nicotine. It helps alleviate symptoms of withdrawal, since it restores normal brain chemistry.

If you are low in phenylalanine or tyrosine, you may feel tired and slow and have trouble concentrating. You may also find it hard to get out of bed in the morning. A dose of either amino acid can help get you mobilized.

Supplements of phenylalanine are available in three different forms:

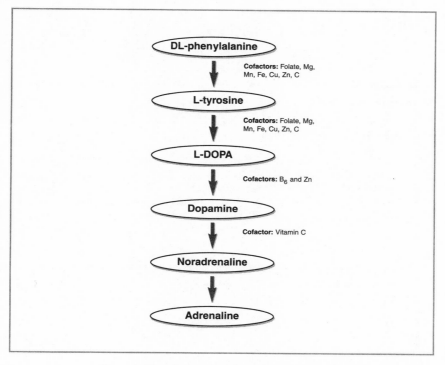

Figure 2. How dopamine and noradrenaline are made from amino acids.

DL-phenylalanine (DLPA), D-phenylalanine, and L-phenylalanine (see Supplement Directory on page 206). The D- and DL-forms have been proven to act as natural painkillers. They enhance the action of endorphins and enkephalins, the natural opiates that reduce pain and produce feelings of well-being, even euphoria. Although some effect is felt within days, the full effect takes a few weeks to build up.

L-phenylalanine combines with vitamin B_6 to produce phenethylamine, the stimulating "love drug" that we find in chocolate (see page 86). One study from 1986 showed that thirty-one of forty depressed patients with low levels of phenythylamine responded well to large doses of L-phenylalanine (up to 14 g a day), making it a very acceptable antidepressant (and, by extension, an antidote for chocolate cravings). In a double-blind study reported in 1979, DLPA (150–200 mg a day) or the antidepressant imipramine

DL-phenylalanine (DLPA)

How it works: Precursor for tyrosine, which converts to dopamine, adrenaline, and noradrenaline.

Positive effects: Enhances mood; promotes energy; relieves pain; controls appetite.

Cautions: Can be too stimulating, causing anxiety, high blood pressure, or insomnia. Should not be taken by people who have the metabolic disease phenylketonuria. Not recommended for those with a history of mania or mental illness.

Dosage: 500–1,000 mg daily on an empty stomach first thing in the morning. Can be repeated later in the day, but not too close to bedtime. Add 25–50 mg of vitamin B_6 and 500 mg of vitamin C daily to enhance its conversion to tyrosine.

was administered to forty depressed patients (twenty in each group) for one month. Both groups had the same positive result, with no statistical difference found between the two groups using both objective and subjective tests.

Taking too much L-phenylalanine or DLPA can lead to overstimulation, resulting in anxiety, insomnia, and hypertension (elevated blood pressure). If this happens, you should then lower the dose, and if symptoms persist, stop taking it altogether. Overall, the best form to use is DLPA, since it is the most comprehensive and least expensive.

The effective dose is usually 500–1,000 mg of DLPA on an empty stomach first thing in the morning. Since everyone has different needs, it's better to start with about half the contents of a 500-mg capsule, taken alone. For quick absorption, open the capsule and put the powder under your tongue. Watch your energy and mood go up. If necessary, you can repeat your dose twice more—mid-morning and mid-afternoon, but not too close to bedtime. You will also need 25–50 mg of vitamin B$_6$ and 500 mg of vitamin C daily to enhance its conversion to tyrosine.

Tyrosine: For Performance

Tyrosine is made in the body from phenylalanine and has the same effects on the brain. It usually acts more rapidly, as it is one step further down the metabolic line. It readily crosses the blood-brain barrier to produce the energizing neurotransmitters dopamine, noradrenaline, and adrenaline. It also is used to make thyroid hormone, the body's energy controller, which manages both metabolic rate and energy production. When your thyroid function is low, so is your energy.

Some people find DLPA more effective than tyrosine for stimulation, but remember that in some people, DLPA is more likely to cause hypertension (high blood pressure). DLPA also differs in its ability to control appetite by releasing CCK, an appetite suppressant made in the gut, and in its action as a pain reliever.

Neither amino acid should be taken with MAOIs (see page 119), antidepressants involving certain food restrictions; by phenylketonurics; by those with malignant melanomas; or by pregnant or breast-feeding women.

Tyrosine has long been known by the military to improve mental and physical performance under stress. Research by the U.S. military found that soldiers given tyrosine in stressful conditions of extreme cold, or while undertaking intense physical activity over prolonged periods of time, showed clear improvements in both mental and physical endurance. More recent research from Holland demonstrates how tyrosine gives you the edge in conditions of stress. A total of twenty-one cadets were put through a demanding one-week military-combat training course; ten of them were given a drink containing 2 g of tyrosine a day, while the remaining eleven were given an identical drink without the tyrosine. Those on tyrosine consistently performed better, both in memorizing the task at hand and in tracking the tasks they had performed.

Since individual sensitivity varies, start with 100 mg or so of tyrosine, even if it means partially emptying out a capsule, and work your way up to your ideal dose. You can take another dose later in the day when your energy is flagging, since DLPA and tyrosine are good, quick energizers. If you are

Tyrosine

How it works: Precursor to the stimulating neurotransmitters dopamine, adrenaline, noradrenaline, and thyroid hormone, thyroxine.

Positive effects: Enhances mood; promotes energy and motivation; supports healthy thyroid function.

Cautions: Hypertension in those susceptible. Should not be taken by people with phenylketonuria, those with melanomas, or pregnant or nursing women. Not recommended for those with a history of mania, unless under a doctor's care.

Dosage: 100–1,000 mg on an empty stomach first thing in the morning to prevent competition from other amino acids. Can be repeated mid-afternoon.

feeling like you need a caffeine boost, open a 500-mg DLPA or tyrosine capsule and put half of the contents under your tongue. It will be quickly absorbed and will give you the kick you want, without the rebound. You may need a whole one, but it's best to try half first. This avoids too much of a rush if you are particularly sensitive to its effects.

In response to regular usage, your brain actually produces more dopamine receptors to "receive" this amino acid. This will raise mood over time in those with depression related to insufficient dopamine receptors, as in reward deficiency syndrome (see page 78). On the other hand, if you don't require it regularly, it's better to use it as needed for a good boost. In clinical practice, we measure the client's amino acid levels and determine if he or she actually needs to supplement. We then recommend supplementation, often in higher doses than those mentioned here, and monitor the patient to be sure that balance is maintained.

OTHER STIMULANTS: BEST OF THE REST

Green Tea

Green tea contains certain important health-giving compounds. Its polyphenols or catechins are potent antioxidants, with cancer-protective and anti-aging effects. Tea also has a blood-thinning effect, similar to that of aspirin. As it turns out, black tea, a fermented form of the same leaf, also contains these compounds, but with proportionately more caffeine along with them. Green tea contains only 20–30 mg of caffeine per cup, as compared to 50 mg in a regular cup of tea, and is consequently less stimulating, even relaxing to many people.

In fact, Asian monks have traditionally used green tea to help keep them awake, but calm, during meditation practice. This is likely due to its content of the amino acid L-theanine (gamma-ethyl-amino-glutamic acid). Mitigating the stimulation of caffeine, within 30–40 minutes of consumption, it produces an increase in alpha brain-wave activity, without drowsiness. The average cup of green tea contains 26–46 mg of theanine, which is available in capsule form as well, in doses of 50–200 mg.

Green Tea

How it works: Contains potent antioxidants and theanine.

Positive effects: Lowers cholesterol and blood pressure; increases HDL, the so-called "good" cholesterol; thins the blood; reduces risk of heart attack, stroke, and cancer; enhances immune function; prevents dental caries and hypertension; aids weight loss by encouraging the body to burn fat. Also produces a state of alert relaxation.

Cautions: Contains caffeine.

Dosage: 1–2 cups a day.

Considering the health benefits, we can count green tea, in moderation (meaning no more than two cups a day), as an acceptable "natural stimulant."

NADH

NADH, or nicotinamide adenine dinucleotide, is a small organic molecule found naturally in every living cell. NADH is necessary for thousands of biochemical reactions within the body and plays a key role in the energy production of cells, particularly in the brain and central nervous system. It stimulates cellular production of the neurotransmitters dopamine, noradrenaline, and serotonin, thereby improving mental clarity, alertness, and concentration. The more NADH a cell has available, the more energy it can produce, and the more efficiently it can perform. It also enhances physical performance and energy. We have found it very useful in the treatment of chronic fatigue syndrome.

NADH

How it works: Stimulates cellular production of the neurotransmitters dopamine, noradrenaline, and serotonin.

Positive effects: Improves mental clarity, cellular memory, alertness, and concentration; is a good antioxidant, and enhances energy and athletic endurance.

Cautions: None.

Dosage: 2.5–10 mg daily, depending on individual requirements.

Coenzyme Q_{10} (Ubiquinone)

No list on natural energizers would be complete without mention of Coenzyme Q_{10}, or CoQ_{10}. Called "ubiquinone" due to its being so ever-present ("ubiquitous"), it is a significant cofactor in driving our engines on a cellular level. From our hearts to our brains, CoQ_{10} helps to convert the nutrients we eat into energy. It is also a potent antioxidant. Another side benefit: it has been shown to stop gums from receding. The recommended dose is 30 mg twice daily, or more if you are taking cholesterol-lowering drugs that deplete CoQ_{10}. Being fat-soluble, it should be taken with a little fat-containing food, such as peanut butter. CoQ_{10} is expensive, but don't just shop price, since the quality is especially important. It is too valuable for your health *not* to have the most effective products.

Coenzyme Q_{10}

How it works: Stimulates cellular production of energy; antioxidant.

Positive effects: Is a good antioxidant; enhances energy and endurance; helps to prevent receding gums.

Cautions: None.

Dosage: 30–300 mg daily, depending on individual requirements.

ACTION PLAN FOR NATURAL STIMULATION

The first steps to maximizing your natural energy and motivation are to reduce your stress level, balance your blood sugar, and avoid or reduce your intake of stimulants to an absolute minimum. A good all-around multivitamin is key. To get started, you'll need to follow the advice in Chapters 3 and 4. Also, Part Three gives you plenty of energy-generating exercises.

Adaptogens are the key supplements for natural, sustained, and healthy stimulation. Asian ginseng can, however, be overstimulating if you have very raised cortisol levels or are exhausted. The same caution does not apply to Siberian ginseng. Licorice can also be overstimulating, so don't supplement it if you are very stressed or exhausted.

The nutrients in the following table are worthy additions to a supplemental program designed to enhance your energy and motivation. Combination formulas are available. It you are taking the supplements individually, start gradually and add new ones only after you have given the products two to three weeks to begin working.

Natural Energizers	Daily Dose
Adaptogenic herbs:	
Siberian ginseng*	100–200 mg
Asian/American ginseng*	100–200 mg
Ashwaganda*	400–900 mg
Rhodiola*	100–200 mg
Reishi mushroom	300–1,000 mg
Amino acids:	
D,L-phenylalanine	100–2,000 mg
Tyrosine	100–2,000 mg
Vitamin:	
Vitamin B$_5$ (pantothenic acid)	100–500 mg
*All amounts given for herbs are for specified standardized extracts.	

So, to sum up, you should take the following to feel alert and energetic:

- A good all-around multivitamin supplying optimal amounts of B vitamins, especially pantothenic acid (vitamin B$_5$) and vitamin C.
- A "stimulant" formula providing Siberian, Asian, or American ginseng, ashwaganda, reishi mushroom, DLPA, and tyrosine.
- Optional licorice, as needed, but only if you are not seriously stressed, and not at night.

For a full natural energy-boost program, see Top Tips in Part Four.

6

Mood Enhancers

The Roots of the Blues

We're all prone to mood shifts, and it's only natural to feel blue from time to time. Occasional bouts of sadness may even help us appreciate the good times. In any case, most of us will bounce back within a short time—hours, days, or even a week or two. For example, when Peter suddenly lost his job of four years, he felt disheartened for a couple of weeks. Then he found a new and even better job, and life was good again. In a similar vein, Stacey was distraught after breaking up with her boyfriend after three years. But with the support of friends, she got over her feelings in a month or two. She was able to put the old relationship in perspective, realized that it ultimately would not have been her best choice, and was soon dating again.

It wasn't quite so simple, though, when Stacey's friend Janet broke up with *her* boyfriend. Janet was in tears for days on end, withdrew from friends and family, and felt like a total failure. Not only did her response seem out of proportion to the event, but she was on a downward spiral, heading toward clinical depression. In fact, Janet always had been more on the "down" side, lacking the joie de vivre of her friend Stacey.

We all fit somewhere within this range, with most of us more or less able to take adversity in stride. But what is it that makes some people less resilient than others? And are there ways to increase our ability to handle the slings and arrows that life flings at us?

We can assure you there are. In this chapter, we'll take a look at what happens in your brain when you're feeling blue. Then we'll cover the anti-depressants commonly prescribed to counter these feelings. Finally, we'll show you how to conquer the blues safely by using a number of natural mood enhancers that can elevate your spirits without the side effects of drugs.

MOOD CHECK

Have you checked yourself out on the Mood Check questionnaire on page 15? Where do you fit on the continuum? Are you happy and content? Clinically depressed? Or somewhere in between?

If you scored within the depressed range, you should start by consulting your physician or health-care practitioner to make sure there is no physical cause for your problems. Then, consult both a psychotherapist and a natural health practitioner. One will deal with psychological issues, while the other will help to find any underlying chemical imbalance that might be causing the problem.

FEED YOUR BRAIN, BEAT THE BLUES

In any case, if you are depressed, don't feel stigmatized. Depression affects one in five people at one time or another in their lives, and it is on the increase worldwide. Moreover, the cause is often biochemical, which is why current treatment approaches include drug therapy as well as psychotherapy.

What is most often overlooked, however, is that mood, behavior, and mental performance all depend on a variety of nutrients that both make up and fuel the brain, nervous system, and neurotransmitters. So a low mood may have less to do with past trauma or a faulty belief system than with deficient nutrients. We've already encountered a number of these, which include vitamins B_3, B_6, folic acid (folate), B_{12}, and C; the minerals zinc and magnesium; essential fatty acids; and the amino acids tryptophan and tyrosine.

Research at King's College Hospital in London, for example, found that 33 percent of those with psychiatric disorders, including depression, were deficient in the B vitamin folate. Other surveys of depressed patients found that many were deficient in iron or B vitamins, especially folate. It seems a shame that with such a simple solution, so many people are suffering needlessly. What is more worrisome is that government dietary surveys show that a large portion of the population doesn't even get the bare minimum, the recommended daily intake (RDI), of these vitamins and minerals in their daily diets. It is no wonder that depression is on the rise!

If poorly nourished, we're less able to cope with life's challenges. Once we're eating the way we should, our mood goes up, and we can handle life's events more resiliently. A good analogy can be found in Dr. Ray Sahelian's book *Mind Boosters*. He compares a happy, healthy mind to a pond with a high water level, representing brain chemicals. There may be many rocks of all shapes and sizes below the tranquil surface. These represent the hurts and traumas that are a part of life. If the water, or brain chemicals, become depleted, the rocks begin to show, and the previously submerged pain comes to the surface. We need to keep the levels topped off for a smooth surface, and a happy mind.

That's not the whole story, however. Taking too much of the wrong substances is just as damaging as failing to take the right ones, with sugar and stimulants topping the list of no-nos. You'll recall how blood-sugar imbalances, often related to excessive sugar, alcohol, or caffeine intake, can stimulate neurotransmitter release and a quick high. Not for long, though: the brain responds to an ongoing use of sugar, as with any drug, by downregulating, leaving you with insufficient feel-good chemicals. There's no doubt that stress, overuse of stimulants, and blood-sugar problems are a major contributor to low moods. Certain medications, including antihistamines, tranquilizers, sleeping pills, narcotics, and recreational drugs, can also interfere with your neurotransmitters, leading to depression.

How, then, do we take on the care and feeding of our brains? We need to start with the key neurotransmitters serotonin and noradrenaline—if these aren't in balance, they can cause depression and low moods. Both anti-depressant drugs and supplements aim to enhance their actions. In fact, a great deal of our information comes from the extensive pharmaceutical research done in the past few decades to develop new antidepressant medications.

Serotonin, tryptophan, and noradrenaline have different roles in countering depression. Depression can be felt as extreme unhappiness or as a lack of drive or motivation, and people can feel more of one or the other, or a mixture of both. Using a psychological test called the Social Adaptation Self-Evaluation Scale, a 1998 study found that a serotonin-enhancing drug had the most effect on self-image and mood, while noradrenaline was more involved in promoting motivation and drive. We will soon see that there are ways to attain these results without taking drugs.

SEROTONIN: THE MOOD NEUROTRANSMITTER

Serotonin is considered the "mood neurotransmitter" that keeps us emotionally and socially stable. It is interesting to note that women seem to have more problems than men in maintaining their serotonin levels. Yes, women are moodier—and this is not a sexist comment, but just a reflection of biological truth, likely due to the interplay between serotonin and the female hormone cycle. This would explain the emotional shifts related to menstrual periods, when many women experience increased moodiness, irritability, and sensitivity to pain. Women who are low in serotonin are likelier to express their anger inwardly, with depression and even suicidal behavior.

Research shows that, in contrast, men who are low in serotonin are often violent and may even engage in dangerous criminal acts. Alcohol and drug abusers also turn out to be low in serotonin. The good news is that we can successfully correct these imbalances by supplying supplements that raise serotonin.

"GOOD MOOD" FOODS:
THE TRYPTOPHAN CONNECTION

Serotonin comes from the essential amino acid tryptophan, which is found in protein-containing foods such as fish, turkey, chicken, cottage cheese, avocados, bananas, and wheat germ. Researchers have found that when they take depressed patients who have improved and deprive them of tryptophan, their depression returns. As we saw in Chapter 2, this has been well demonstrated by research at Oxford University's Department of Psychiatry. Women with a history of depression were divided into two groups and were given a diet excluding or including tryptophan under double-blind conditions (that is, neither the subjects nor the researchers knew who received which diet). At the end of the experiment, ten out of fifteen women on the tryptophan-free diet were significantly depressed, while no one on the tryptophan diet had any problem at all. When the participants in the deprived group were given a diet containing tryptophan, their depression lifted.

In general, giving tryptophan to people with depression has been beneficial, although some trials have not found that it had a significant effect when compared with a placebo. One possible explanation is that, without sufficient vitamins B_3 and B_6, tryptophan can be processed along a different chemical pathway, turning into a substance called kynurenine instead of serotonin (see Figure 3). We can also supplement with an amino acid called 5-hydroxytryptophan (5-HTP), which is one step closer to turning into serotonin, explained in more detail on page 125.

NORADRENALINE: BE REWARDED

The neurotransmitter noradrenaline provides us with feelings of both motivation and pleasure. Derived from dopamine, noradrenaline is involved with positive stress states such as being in love, the thrill of music and dancing, and other exhilarating and stimulating pursuits. As we mentioned in Chapter 5, some people inherit a gene that makes them deficient in these neurotransmitters, leaving them more prone to depression. They also

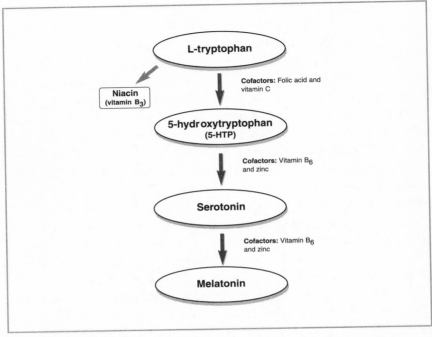

Figure 3. How the essential amino acid tryptophan can transform into serotonin and melatonin.

crave stimulation from sugar, coffee, stress, and alcohol. With reward deficiency syndrome (RDS), people have a hard time feeling good, or "rewarded," under normal conditions. They can enhance their mood and motivation, and even reduce cravings for the addictive substances, by taking the precursor amino acids tyrosine and phenylalanine. These amino acids convert to dopamine with the help of vitamin cofactors such as vitamin B_6 and folic acid. You don't have to have RDS to benefit from these nutrients, however. Many people are deficient for various reasons and feel better once levels are normalized.

So much for how your brain stays happy. Now we'll take a look at the antidepressants commonly used to chase the blues away.

Antidepressants: The Pros and Cons

Researchers began developing a number of synthetic drugs for the treatment of depression in the 1950s—and they took off in a big way. At the time, they were seen as a breakthrough. Now, a large variety of antidepressant medications is available. Distinguished by how they affect the balance and function of specific neurotransmitters, they fall into four principal classes: the tricyclic drugs, the selective serotonin reuptake inhibitors (SSRIs), the monoamine oxidase inhibitors (MAOIs), and the noradrenaline reuptake inhibitor drugs (NARIs). There are other antidepressant drugs that are chemically distinct both from these types and from one another.

Antidepressants have helped many desperate people live happier lives. However, these powerful medications have also been greatly overprescribed. There is plenty of good scientific evidence that natural products will often work just as well and without the side effects.

The various types of antidepressants differ in their mechanisms of action and side effects. However, they all have several things in common: They are effective in reducing depressive symptoms in 50 to 80 percent of those who use them. They may take from four to six weeks to produce their full effects, although side effects and changes in mood can occur much sooner.

THE TRICYCLICS

Competing only with the problematic MAO inhibitors, tricyclics dominated the market for some twenty years. Used less frequently now, they work in various ways to affect the actions of noradrenaline and serotonin. There are a number of frightening downsides to these drugs as revealed below.

Downside of Tricyclics

Tricyclics can induce drowsiness, dizziness, heart palpitations, dry mouth, blurred vision, confusion, weight gain, sweating, rashes, nausea, constipation or diarrhea, difficulty with urination, impotence or impaired erection in men, inhibited orgasm in women, nightmares, and anxiety.

SSRIS: PROZAC WORKS,
BUT THE SIDE EFFECTS ARE DEPRESSING

As we now know, serotonin, "the civilizing neurotransmitter," plays a vital role in mood, memory, appetite, sleep, pain perception, and sexual desire. Serotonin reuptake inhibitors, or SSRIs, block the neuron's reabsorption of serotonin. This makes more of the neurotransmitter available, with a resulting elevation in mood. Currently prescribed SSRIs include fluoxetine (Prozac), fluvoxamine (Luvox), paroxetine (Paxil), sertraline (Zoloft), and citalopram (Celexa).

While the SSRIs don't have the same side effects as the tricyclics, they do bring their own problems. First, they often compromise libido and sexual performance in most men and women. Second, they are not euphoriants, but rather mood stabilizers, and even mood flatteners. They often limit the highs along with the lows, and many people taking them end up with a zombielike lack of emotion, as well as a host of other side effects (see the downsides below).

Here is what one Prozac user's husband describes:

> My wife was on Prozac. It led her to have an "I don't give a darn" attitude about important things, and she had stomach pain the entire time she was on it. She then went off Prozac and started on St. John's wort. The stomach problems went away the day she stopped Prozac. Now that she's on St. John's wort, her depression hasn't returned. She is relaxed and cares again about the important things in her life.

And here is what Jan, another user of SSRIs, has to say:

> I've suffered from "the blues" all my life. I took the antidepressant Zoloft, 100 mg twice a day. It worked, but it was expensive and I couldn't stand the side effects. I am also not sure I liked the leveling off of all my emotions! So, a month ago I began substituting St. John's wort, two tablets at night instead of the Zoloft. I'm very happy with the results. I no longer have debilitating PMS, either.

Downsides of Prozac and Other SSRIs

Prozac and other SSRIs can compromise libido and sexual performance in men and women; can "flatten" moods to the point of zombielike emotionlessness; can bring on forty-five other side effects, including nausea, nervousness, insomnia, headache, tremors, anxiety, drowsiness, dry mouth, excessive sweating, and diarrhea; and can have long-term withdrawal effects that look a lot like the above-mentioned side effects.

THE MONOAMINE OXIDASE INHIBITORS (MAOIS): FOOD WARNINGS

The monoamine oxidase inhibitors, or MAOIs, such as phenelzine sulfate (Nardil) and tranylcypromine sulfate (Parnate), work by reducing the quantity of the enzyme MAO (monoamine oxidase) within the synapses. Since MAO ordinarily breaks down neurotransmitters, its reduction leads to higher adrenaline and dopamine levels. MAOIs can produce a dangerous elevation in blood pressure, called the "cheese effect," if the patient also takes decongestants, antihistamines, or foods containing the amino acid tyramine, such as aged cheese or red wine.

Downside of MAOIs

Taking MAOIs with decongestants, antihistamines, or foods containing tyramine, such as cheese or red wine, can cause dangerously high blood pressure.

OTHER ANTIDEPRESSANTS

There are some antidepressants that appear to affect neurotransmitter activity but don't fit in the above categories: bupropion (Wellbutrin), trazodone (Desyrel), venlafaxine (Effexor), and nefazdone (Serzone).

All this said, there is a role for medications as well as for herbs in psychiatric treatment. There are circumstances when one or the other is called for, and there are situations when they are needed in combination. However, the synthetic pharmaceutical medications should be reserved for those times when their benefits outweigh their downsides. During my years of psychiatric practice, I have learned that natural supplements should be the first line of treatment. Their more gentle actions are often all that is needed to resolve the imbalances leading to depression, as you will see in the section that follows.

Nature's Blues Busters

Many people prone to depression have found that they can control their moods very well with natural supplements, which don't have the side effects of antidepressant drugs. The information that follows will help you to know which ones to take and the anticipated effects.

While SSRIs tend to increase the supply of neurotransmitters by inhibiting reuptake or by preventing their breakdown, nutritional supplements provide the basic "construction materials." If your mood problems are due to a deficiency in the materials that make up the neurotransmitters, then simply inhibiting their reuptake won't solve your problem in the long run. That is one reason why the drugs often stop working after awhile.

The key mood-enhancing herbs and nutrients are:

- St. John's wort.
- L-tryptophan and 5-HTP.
- Phenylalanine and tyrosine (see Chapter 5).
- SAMe and TMG.
- Omega-3 fats—EPA and DHA.
- B vitamins, vitamin C, and zinc.

Figure 4 shows how our brains make and maintain the right balance of neurotransmitters that enhance our moods and keep us motivated. Ensuring an optimal intake of these nutrients is the best way to stay happy.

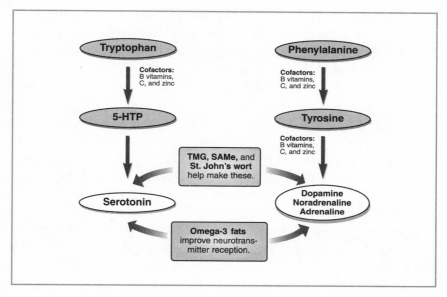

Figure 4. How mood-enhancing nutrients keep us motivated and happy.

ST. JOHN'S WORT: WONDER WEED

Imagine an antidepressant that is as effective as prescription drugs but has mild side effects, if any, and even boosts libido. Sound like a fantasy? It's not. You've just met St. John's wort, an herb taken by many thousands of people every day. In fact, in Europe, *Hypericum perforatum* is prescribed by doctors five times as often as Prozac.

Animal studies show that St. John's wort inhibits the reuptake of serotonin and possibly also of dopamine and noradrenaline. It appears to act like both SSRIs and tricyclic antidepressants, but without their side effects.

A 1996 review of twenty-three randomized clinical trials on St. John's wort, involving a total of 1,700 people, showed an equivalent response to antidepressants with minimal side effects. At a dose of 300 mg a day of a 0.3 percent hypericin extract, St. John's wort appears to help those with mild to moderate depression. There is even some evidence that doubling this dose can help those with severe depression. St. John's wort is also useful in calming your nerves and in helping you to sleep more soundly.

While hypericin has been generally accepted as the active antidepressant ingredient and is used as the marker in standardization, there is newer evidence that the hyperforin may actually be the more active antidepressant compound. As a result, you may begin to see more St. John's wort products on the market that are standardized to hyperforin, in addition to the usual hypericin.

Because St. John's wort was originally believed to work through MAO inhibition (see page 119), some articles still list the MAOI food restrictions. However, it is now quite clear that St. John's wort in normal doses does not have this effect. But there are a number of cautions associated with the

St. John's Wort Versus Antidepressant Drugs

St. John's wort:

- Its side effects are not nearly as severe or frequent.
- Mixing it with alcohol doesn't lead to adverse reactions, as with the pharmaceutical antidepressants.
- It is not addictive.
- It does not produce withdrawal symptoms when you stop.
- It does not produce habituation or the need for increased dosages to maintain its effects.
- It can be easily stopped and restarted without requiring a long build-up period.
- It enhances sleep and dreaming.
- Unlike SSRIs, it does not inhibit sex drive—and can actually enhance it.
- It does not make you sleepy in the daytime. Experiments show that it can enhance alertness and driving reaction time.
- According to one report, the annual rate of death by overdose on antidepressant drugs is 30.1 per 1 million prescriptions. No one has ever died from an overdose of St. John's wort.

herb, as you'll see below. To put it into perspective, though: Most of the cautions here relate to a rather small minority of the population. Also, many common drugs *and even grapefruit juice* will have similar effects, since they activate the same liver enzymes that St. John's wort does.

St. John's Wort

How it works: Appears to inhibit reuptake of the neurotransmitters serotonin, noradrenaline, and dopamine; enhances GABA activity as well.

Positive effects: Enhances mood; acts as an antidepressant; combats anxiety in most people; helps regulate sleep.

Cautions: May cause allergic reactions, rashes, gastrointestinal problems, or sun sensitivity in susceptible individuals. Can cause anxiety or insomnia if taken too close to bedtime. Can reduce the potency of protease inhibitors (taken as treatment for AIDS) or cyclosporin (an immunosuppressant taken by organ transplant patients), digoxin (heart medication), or even, possibly, birth control pills (with two recent reported cases of pregnancy). St. John's wort has not been researched sufficiently to recommend it for use during pregnancy or nursing. If combined with 5-HTP (see page 125), there is the possibility of serotonin syndrome—headache, an increase in body temperature, and heavy sweating. Seek medical help if this occurs.

Dosage: 300 mg daily of an extract of 0.3 percent hypericin, starting with one or two capsules or tablets in the morning with breakfast. If there is no change in mood after a week, add a third dose at lunch, for a total of 900 mg daily. You can also take it as two doses of 450 mg each, or take your entire daily dose in the morning, since the herb stays in the body for a long time (about 24 hours) before being broken down.

L-TRYPTOPHAN: LOST AND FOUND

We've already read about L-tryptophan. But what about taking it as a supplement? A once popular over-the-counter treatment for depression and insomnia, L-tryptophan was banned in the United States by the Food and Drug Administration in 1989, after a contaminated batch from Japan caused a serious illness called "eosinophilia myalgia syndrome" (EMS). Despite the fact that the exact cause of this outbreak was determined to be due to specific contamination, the FDA persisted in their declaration that L-tryptophan itself was unsafe. It is interesting to note that tryptophan continues to be available in infant formulas and in concentrated food formulas for those too ill to be fed normally.

One can at least speculate that the explanation for such an obvious inconsistency can be found in the enormous financial and political influence

---

L-tryptophan

How it works: Raw material or precursor for the neurotransmitter serotonin.

Positive effects: Elevates mood; promotes relaxation, emotional stability, healthy sleep-wake patterns, deep sleep, dreaming, and creative imagination.

Cautions: May cause nausea, headaches, constipation, and other gastrointestinal problems in certain people, especially in high doses. It should not be taken during pregnancy, with MAO inhibitors, or in cases of the autoimmune disease lupus. It is inadvisable to take both tryptophan and SSRI antidepressants except under medical guidance.

Dosage: 500–1,000 mg two to three times daily for the treatment of depression or insomnia. Best absorbed away from protein and with a carbohydrate snack. Take a B-complex vitamin that contains 50 mg of B_6, and a minimum of 15 mg of zinc. If used for insomnia, take the dose one hour before bedtime.

---

of pharmaceuticals companies, which would rather have you buy their prescription drugs for depression and insomnia. So perhaps the politics of prejudice against self-administered supplements played a role here.

L-tryptophan, which is currently available only by prescription, usually comes in 500-mg capsules. The recommended dose is 500–1,000 mg, or up to 2,000 mg daily. You can take 500 mg or so in the morning, and 500–1,500 mg one hour before bedtime if you need help in falling asleep. The enzyme tryptophan hydroxylase, which converts tryptophan into 5-HTP (see below), depends on folic acid and vitamin C. 5-HTP is turned into serotonin, with the aid of the cofactors biotin, vitamin B_6, and zinc, and the enzyme 5-HTP carboxylase. Make sure you are getting enough of these cofactors by supplementing with a high-potency multivitamin. Also, a carbohydrate snack, such as fruit, acts as a vehicle to transport it into the brain. Since other amino acids or proteins will compete for the same space, don't take tryptophan with protein-rich foods.

5-HTP (5-HYDROXYTRYPTOPHAN): OUT OF AFRICA

In 1995, 5-HTP—the metabolite of tryptophan, a step further along in the metabolic pathway—became available as an extract from seeds of the African shrub *Griffonia simplicifolia*. Like L-tryptophan, it is converted into serotonin, inducing relaxation, elevated mood, and sleep. It may be even more useful than tryptophan, because much of the tryptophan we eat is processed along different biochemical pathways. 5-HTP is a direct precursor of serotonin and also enters the brain more easily. Unlike tryptophan, it can be taken with food and other supplements, including amino acids, with no interference. It still needs vitamin B_6 as a cofactor for conversion to serotonin.

Not surprisingly, results in treating depression with 5-HTP have proven more effective than with tryptophan. For example, a double-blind trial headed by Dr. Poldinger at the Basel University of Psychiatry gave thirty-four depressed patients 300 mg of 5-HTP and twenty-nine patients fluvoxamine (Luvox), an SSRI antidepressant. Each patient was assessed for his or her degree of depression using the widely accepted Hamilton Rating Scale, plus his or her own subjective self-assessment. At the end of the six weeks, both groups showed a significant improvement in their depression. However, those patients taking 5-HTP experienced a greater improvement in each of the four criteria assessed—depression, anxiety, insomnia, and physical symptoms—as well as the patients' self-assessments. 5-HTP had outperformed the best antidepressant. Given that 5-HTP is less expensive and has significantly fewer side effects, it is extraordinary that it is almost never prescribed by psychiatrists.

The dose of 5-HTP is one-tenth that of L-tryptophan. It is available in both 50- and 100-mg capsules. For anxiety or depression, the dose is 50–200 mg a day, taken in divided doses. Some people report drowsiness if they take 5-HTP during the day, so use caution to determine your best daytime dose. In fact, especially if you're having trouble sleeping, you can take 50–200 mg of the daily dose at bedtime. Since there are few studies on the long-term effects, it is best taken for a month or two at a time only, with a few weeks off before restarting.

5-HTP (5-hydroxytryptophan)

How it works: Direct precursor for the neurotransmitter serotonin.

Positive effects: Induces relaxation; elevates mood and sleep; suppresses appetite; promotes healthy sleep-wake patterns and emotional stability, dreaming, and creative imagination.

Cautions: Some people report nausea, anxiety, and agitation at very high doses. Rarely, sensitive individuals may feel anxious at even normal doses, in which case they should stop. Do not take 5-HTP with SSRI antidepressants except under medical guidance.

Dosage: For daytime use, 50–100 mg two to three times daily. For sleep, 50–200 mg one hour before bedtime. Take about 50 mg a day of vitamin B_6 as a cofactor.

PHENYLALANINE AND TYROSINE: DYNAMIC DUO

These natural mood boosters have already been covered extensively in Chapter 5. For a complete rundown on them and essential information on possible downsides, doses, and so on, see pages 102 to 106. Phenylalanine and tyrosine are amino acid precursors to noradrenaline, adrenaline, and dopamine.

Phenylalanine is converted to tyrosine, which is then converted to dopamine, and then to noradrenaline. They require as cofactors the vitamins niacin, B_6, B_{12}, folic acid, and C, plus the minerals zinc, magnesium, copper, iron, and manganese. The most effective form of phenylalanine for mood enhancement is DLPA, which has proven as effective as tricyclic antidepressants.

Most of the research on people's moods is conducted by pharmaceutical companies while they are developing new drugs. Experiments are first run on laboratory animals. Then people suffering from depression are recruited as their test subjects. As a result, we don't have much "official" information on the effects of these substances in "normal" people, who want to take products simply to boost their mood. But our own clinical experience shows us that these are great mood boosters, even when there is no obvious problem.

SAMe: TURNING ON THE LIGHTS

Recently, there has been a great deal of media attention focused on the natural compound SAMe (s-adenosyl-methionine), pronounced "Sammy." A new "convert" to SAMe, thirty-five-year-old Marisa, shares the following experience:

> I had been feeling just "blah" for what seemed like years. I read about St. John's wort and took it for a few months, 300 mg, three times daily. I felt somewhat better, but something was still missing. Then I added SAMe, 400 mg a day. It's like someone turned on the lights. I felt like a kid again, playing, being happy, and not as burdened as I had become.

For those of you with no mood problems, but just wanting to feel a little high, you can expect a similar experience. An appropriate dose, discussed below, on an empty stomach can put a spring in your step, a sparkle in your eye, and a grin on your face.

Placebo-controlled, double-blind studies show that SAMe is equal or superior to antidepressants and works faster, most often within a few days (most pharmaceutical antidepressants may take three to six weeks to take effect), with no significant side effects. Instead, SAMe has *side benefits:* It is an effective treatment for degenerative joint disease, fibromyalgia, and liver problems. According to one comprehensive review of all the studies, 92 percent of depressive patients responded to SAMe, while only 85 percent responded to antidepressant medications.

If you stop taking SAMe suddenly, you'll experience no withdrawal reaction—a common pitfall when antidepressants are stopped abruptly. SAMe also protects your liver, in contrast to the potential liver damage triggered by some tricyclic antidepressants.

Except for the adrenal and pineal glands, the liver contains the most SAMe of any body organ. In the body, the liver depends on SAMe for regeneration, detoxification, bile production, and the essential biochemical processes of both methylation and the production of glutathione, the liver's natural antioxidant. SAMe aids the liver in neutralizing toxins, carcinogens, and free radicals. This slows the aging process, including that of the brain.

That's not all. Research shows that SAMe treats the fatigue, inflammation, and pain associated with fibromyalgia, a puzzling and hard-to-treat condition. Patients have reported significant benefits from taking 400–800 mg of SAMe daily, including improved sleep, reduced fatigue and pain, and enhanced mood. All in all, quite a remarkable nutrient!

How much should you take? SAMe should be taken on an empty stomach, preferably one hour between meals, and at least 20 minutes away from other supplements. If you experience nausea or gastrointestinal problems, reduce the dose and take it with meals although the food will somewhat cut its potency.

Start with 200 mg once or twice daily, which will often be enough. If you don't see results in a few days, you can gradually increase the dose by

200 mg every three days, up to a maximum of 400 mg four times daily (1,600 mg). Then, once your mood feels stable, you can gradually reduce your intake to a lower maintenance dose. In general, the longer SAMe is used, the better the results.

To enhance production of the SAMe precursor, methionine, you need to take its cofactors vitamins B_6 (50 mg), B_{12} (1,000 mcg), and folic acid (800 mcg). Rather than taking the cofactors along with SAMe, they can simply be taken as part of your daily multivitamin regimen.

A limiting factor in SAMe's use has been its high cost, especially at doses as high as 1,600 mg a day. Don't skimp on quality, though. Purchase it from a reputable company, in pharmaceutical-grade enteric-coated tablets. Refrigerate it whenever possible. In comparing products by potency and price, look for the amount of active ingredient on the label. For example, 200 mg of s-adenosyl-methionine butanedisulfonate provides only 50 percent or 100 mg of SAMe.

A word of caution: Though this effect is not reported in the literature, higher doses can cause irritability, anxiety, or insomnia in some people. In this case, lower the dose, but if the effect continues, stop taking it. By the same token, SAMe's antidepressant activity may trigger a manic phase in individuals with bipolar disorder, so they should not take SAMe unless under medical supervision. The same cautions apply to the use of TMG (below).

TRIMETHYLGLYCINE (TMG): MORE OF THE SAMe

The body can also make SAMe directly from trimethylglycine (TMG), which is much less expensive. While it has not been as extensively researched as SAMe, the fact that it is a direct precursor of SAMe would predict that its effect would be similar.

TMG is also known as "glycine betaine," not to be confused with "betaine hydrochloride," which is used to help increase stomach acid. TMG turns homocysteine, a substance toxic to the heart, into SAMe and methionine. This process also yields DMG (dimethylglycine), a well-known performance and energy enhancer, which thus doubles TMG's benefits. DMG

SAMe (s-adenosyl-methionine) and TMG (trimethylglycine)

How they work: Naturally occurring molecules, essential in the manufacture of neurotransmitters.

Positive effects: Enhance neurotransmitter activity; act as natural mood enhancers and stimulants.

Cautions: Higher doses may lead to irritability, anxiety, insomnia, and nausea. SAMe's antidepressant activity may lead to the manic phase in individuals with bipolar disorder (manic depression), so they should be monitored carefully.

Dosage: 200 mg of SAMe once or twice daily, between meals, increasing gradually to a maximum of 1,600 mg a day if needed; *or* 500–3,000 mg of TMG once or twice daily.

can also be used, generally in sublingual tablets that dissolve quickly under the tongue.

Extracted from sugar beets, TMG is also found in broccoli and spinach. Except for the cautions listed above, it has no reported side effects other than brief muscle-tension headaches, and only if it is taken in large quantities without food. Optimal doses needed to raise SAMe are 1,000–3,000 mg per day. In a combination formula, 250–500 mg is enough.

An important point is that, unlike many other natural and synthetic antidepressants, SAMe and TMG are safe to take during pregnancy and nursing. There are also no reported negative interactions with other medications, such as antidepressants. This makes them particularly useful for elderly people who are often on a variety of medications and are also more sensitive to side effects. SAMe can be used safely with other natural supplements, too, including St. John's wort.

OMEGA-3 BRAIN FATS: THE FISH CONNECTION

You've learned how important the omega-3 fatty acids are for health and, as it turns out, for happiness. The omega-3 fatty acids, EPA and DHA, are found in fatty, carnivorous fish such as herring, mackerel, tuna, and salmon. In countries where there is higher fish consumption, there is a lower rate of depression. Also, diets and drugs that severely lower cholesterol tend to exacerbate omega-3 deficiency, causing depression, whereas supplementing omega-3 fish oils has proven effective in elevating mood. There is also a correlation between the incidence of depression and heart disease, and both are associated with omega-3 fat deficiency. (For a more complete discussion of the research on the omega-3 fats, see page 38.)

To ensure an optimal intake of the essential omega-3s, eat fatty fish three times a week. Otherwise, take an omega-3 fish oil supplement providing 500–1,000 mg of EPA plus DHA, daily. Most fish oil supplements provide around 400 mg of EPA plus DHA, so you'll need two a day. If you are vegan or vegetarian, eat one tablespoon of flaxseeds a day and one tablespoon of flaxseed oil.

EPA and DHA

How they work: Build material for neuron membranes and neurotransmitter receptor sites; enhance neural transmission; increase serotonin levels.

Positive effects: Improve learning, memory, and mood in depression, bipolar disorder, and dyslexia.

Cautions: None.

Dosage: 500–1,000 mg a day, as a combined EPA/DHA fish oil supplement, or eat fatty fish three times a week as an antioxidant.

B VITAMINS AND MINERALS: FOOD FOR THOUGHT

Some of your brain's best friends, the B vitamins, have many roles to play in ensuring optimal brain function. They are vital for delivering oxygen to the brain and protecting it from harmful oxidants. They also help turn glucose into energy within brain cells and help to keep neurotransmitters in circulation. Vitamins B_6, B_{12}, and folic acid are most important in terms of enhancing mood.

Vitamin B_6 (Pyridoxine)

Vitamin B_6 has an important role in brain function: it's essential for the manufacture of neurotransmitters, such as the conversion of tryptophan into serotonin, and tyrosine into dopamine. As you learned, a deficiency in these important neurotransmitters can cause depression and other problems. One study showed that about one-fifth of the people with depression who took part were deficient in vitamin B_6. We suggest you take 20–100 mg a day.

Vitamin B_{12} (Cyanocobalamin)

Essential for the health of nerve cells, the usual dose of vitamin B_{12} is 10–1,000 mcg per day. Since there is a decrease with age in a stomach substance called "intrinsic factor," which is required for the absorption of vitamin B_{12}, deficiency of B_{12} is a major cause of mental deterioration and confusion in older people. They may benefit from taking much higher amounts, such as 1,000 mcg daily, and from taking a form that is easier to absorb, such as tablets or liquid that dissolve under the tongue.

Folic Acid (Folate)

Like vitamin B_{12}, folic acid is essential for oxygen delivery to the brain. Deficiency in either results in anemia. In high doses, folic acid has been shown to substantially lessen depression and symptoms of schizophrenia. You need about 400 mcg daily.

It is important to remember that B vitamins should be taken in combination to avoid possible side effects. For example, too much vitamin B_6 on its own can cause neurological problems. If you want to supplement a specific B vitamin, take it along with a multivitamin containing all the other B vitamins for balance.

ACTION PLAN FOR A NATURAL MOOD LIFT

From a biochemical perspective, here's what to do to enhance your mood, but do bear in mind that low moods can be due to psychological factors as well. These are discussed in Chapter 15.

- Start with the Natural High Basics diet and supplements, including fish or flaxseed oil or a regular dietary intake of fish and/ or flaxseeds. Your basic supplement program should include a high-strength multivitamin and vitamin C, supplying optimal amounts of B vitamins.
- Balance your blood-sugar levels by avoiding sugar and stimulants and eating slow-releasing carbohydrates such as whole grains and fruit. Remember that a high-carbohydrate meal can make you drowsy, as can low blood sugar.

Once these basics are met, and you still need a boost, there are specific supplement recommendations. Some mood-enhancing supplement formulas combine many of these nutrients. The ideal doses are less when combined than when taken in isolation. Remember, the supplements listed below should be taken one (or two) at a time to start. Give the products a few weeks to begin working and only then try to add new ones. Do not start by taking them all together.

- 5-HTP: Daily dose is 50 mg in the morning, and 50–100 mg at bedtime to raise your serotonin levels. It is a calming, mood-enhancing amino acid. If you get drowsy from the morning dose, which is rare, take the entire dose of 50–200 mg at bedtime. If it's too activating, as happens with some people, switch to the prescription form, L-tryptophan (which may also be activating in the rare individual).
- St. John's wort: 300 mg daily of an extract of 0.3 percent hypericin, starting with one or two capsules or tablets in the morn-

ing with breakfast. If there is no change after a week, add a third dose at lunch. You can also take it as two doses of 450 mg each, or take your entire daily dose in the morning. If combining with 5-HTP, start with one capsule and build up slowly, since there is the *theoretical* possibility of serotonin syndrome. This happens when you have an overload of serotonin. Its symptoms are headache, increased body temperature, and excessive perspiration. If this should occur, seek medical help immediately. Don't worry too much, though. We have not seen or heard of such a case yet.

Taking St. John's wort too close to bedtime can interfere with sleep in some people. Others find it relaxing. Available in tinctures as well, it can be taken by dropper. Since the tinctures are not standardized, read the label for the dose. You may need a few weeks to feel the full effect, so be patient.

- If you tend to be low in energy and unmotivated first thing in the morning, despite sufficient sleep, 100–1,000 mg of tyrosine or

Mood Enhancers	Daily Dose
L-tryptophan	500–3,000 mg
5-HTP	50–300 mg
St. John's wort	300–900 mg
Tyrosine	100–2,000 mg
DLPA	100–2,000 mg
SAMe	200–1,600 mg
TMG	250–500 mg
Vitamin B_3 (niacin)	40–100 mg
Vitamin B_5 (pantothenic acid)	100–500 mg
Vitamin B_6 (pyridoxine)	20–50 mg
Vitamin B_{12} (cyanocobalamin)	10–1,000 mcg
Folic acid	400–800 mcg

DL-phenylalanine should pick you up. You can gradually increase to 2,000 mg if necessary.

- SAMe is next if you still need a mood boost. Take 200 mg twice daily on an empty stomach. If you haven't felt an improvement in a few days, increase gradually, up to 400 mg four times daily. Most often, 400 mg daily is sufficient. In general, the longer SAMe is used, the more beneficial the results. Once you reach an effective level, you can start cutting back to an optimum maintenance dose. Alternatively, take 250–500 mg of TMG or DMG. SAMe does not mix well with other products, so either take it separately or replace it with TMG.

So, to sum up, you should take the following to lift your mood:

- A good all-around multivitamin supplying optimal amounts of B vitamins (see Chapter 3).
- Either a EPA/DHA-rich fish oil supplement or fish three times a week in a meal. The fish oils must be taken separately since they cannot be combined in a tablet.
- A mood-booster formula providing many of the nutrients shown above (see Supplement Directory on page 206).

For a full natural mood-lift program, see Top Tips in Part Four.

Mind and Memory Boosters

Time bears away all things, even our minds.
VIRGIL 70 B.C.

Losing Your Mind?

It happens to all of us: our concentration becomes fuzzy, our minds slow down, and we struggle, wracking our brains to pin names to faces or recall schedules and phone numbers.

In a vain effort to kick-start our minds, we find ourselves turning more and more to coffee, sugar, and other stimulants. As we saw in Chapter 5, this isn't much of a solution. But we want to be sharp and clear-headed. With a good memory and active mind, we can generate ideas, solve problems, and generally feel in charge of our lives. Then we begin to worry if this is the price we must pay for having abused our minds and bodies— with too much stress, bad food, booze, and drugs—or is it just the inevitable result of aging?

In fact, declining mental function, which often starts to become noticeable in a person's forties, is not inevitable. The good news is, you *can* get your mind in gear again—and even make it work better than before. We'll show you how. By the end of this chapter, you may well find that full mental clarity is within your grasp. But first, let's identify where your problems lie. You may want to turn back to the Memory Check questionnaire on page 16 to remind yourself (in case you forgot!).

YOU MUST REMEMBER THIS . . .

Do you sometimes *know* you know something, but fail to make the connections? For example, when you recognize a face but can't remember the name that goes with it? The reason for this is that memories are held not in one, but in several brain cells that join together to form a network. For a memory to be encoded, it must enter the cells by the mechanism of your seeing, hearing, or doing something. This results in three kinds of memory—visual, auditory, and kinesthetic. If you want to be sure to remember something, you need to bring all these into play and involve the maximum number of brain cells. To remember a telephone number, look at it, repeat it to yourself aloud, and punch the numbers on the phone several times. That's the best way to connect.

Let's take a look at the whole picture—how memory loss is affecting us as we age. Then we'll see what can be done about it. As it happens, there's quite a lot we can do.

The Big Fadeout: Age and Stress

In most people, 20 percent of brain cells die over a lifetime. When you reach seventy, your brain will have shrunk by 10 percent. These changes are often accompanied by a gradual loss of control of the complex orchestra of hormones and neurotransmitters that keeps you on the ball. The result is diminished brain power—slower memory retrieval, reduced sex drive, poor motivation, slower thinking and learning, low energy, poor motivation, and fewer highs.

According to the drug companies, memory decline is becoming a massive and widespread problem. Although it is a much less severe condition, *age-related cognitive decline (ARCD)* affects many more people than Alzheimer's disease. "We believe at least 4 million people in the United Kingdom suffer from this," says Dr. Paul Williams of GlaxoSmithKline, a pharmaceutical company that has been developing drugs to enhance memory and mental performance. A 1994 survey found that 56 percent of respondents report frequently losing things at age forty-five, while 75 percent did so at age seventy-five. Remembering names was a problem for 46 percent at age forty-five, increasing to over 50 percent at age seventy-five.

So widespread is the epidemic of ARCD that the pharmaceutical industry has developed more than 140 different "smart" pills to combat it, making them the tenth largest class of drugs being researched according to a report in *The Economist* magazine. Even larger than the market for Alzheimer's is the growing market for drugs to treat the new problem of ARCD. Just as attention deficit disorder (ADD) was taken seriously once it was classified as a real disease, giving a name to this gradual loss of memory allows doctors to prescribe smart drugs to those whose memories need a boost. As you'll see in this chapter, we recommend smart *nutrients*—our natural mind and memory boosters—instead.

Even more worrisome is the fact that Alzheimer's disease is on the increase. What could be worse than losing your mind when your body still has many years to run? Yet that is precisely what happens to one in ten people over the age of sixty-five, and one in two over age eighty-five. With our rapidly aging population, by the year 2030, 20 percent of people over age sixty-five will have Alzheimer's disease. The stress caused by Alzheimer's, both to the victim and the family, is immense. For many people falling down the slippery slope of Alzheimer's, the first signs are depression, irritability, confusion, and forgetfulness. While its causes are multidetermined, and some are yet to be revealed, there are still some preventive measures we can take to slow its progress.

Stress-Related Memory Loss

Stress has an enormous impact on our memories, too. A *mild* dose of stress can actually *stimulate* memory and mental alertness, but long-term stress is definitely bad news: it puts too much of the hormone cortisol into circulation, and this literally damages the brain. Elevated levels of cortisol have been linked to poorer memory and a shrinking of the brain's memory processing center—the *hippocampus.*

When you were a student, did you stress yourself out studying night after night for exams, only to perform badly on the day of the test? Mental burnout caused by prolonged stress can interfere with memory recall. According to Stanford University researcher Robert Sapolsky, after only two weeks of exposure to stress-induced cortisol levels, dendrites—the "arms" of brain cells that reach out and connect with other cells—begin to shrivel up.

It all sounds pretty grim. But luckily, you can actually reverse all these trends, from damage by stress to age-related memory loss. Short of a dip in the Fountain of Youth, here's how.

REVERSING MEMORY LOSS

Dr. Sapolsky found that when you reduce stress—and, in turn, reduce cortisol levels—the dendrites grow back! You need to cut back on stimulants like tea, coffee, or cigarettes, and opt for natural alternatives, such as ginseng, which halts the overproduction of cortisol and improves the ability of the adrenal glands to respond to stress (see Chapter 5).

Take action now. Neither age-related memory loss nor Alzheimer's disease is inevitable—you can build new brain cells at any age. Research clearly shows that healthy, well-educated elderly people can maintain optimal mental function, with no decline and with no increase in the rate of brain shrinkage, even after age sixty-five. It's a "use it or lose it" situation, and the steps you need to take to keep all your marbles are the same as those needed to maximize your memory and mental alertness. So, whether you are twenty or sixty years old, the time to act is now. The program revolves around diet, exercise, reducing stress levels, and taking specific nutrients that boost mental function.

Eat a diet high in antioxidant nutrients and supplement with nutrients such as vitamins A, C, E, and selenium and zinc (for more on this, see Chapter 3) to neutralize free radicals. These are toxic molecules formed by normal metabolic oxidative reactions and by chemicals that we ingest and inhale from our environment. Without a good supply of protective antioxidants, free radicals can damage your brain cells.

By the same token, be sure you eat plenty of fats for the brain. Omega-3 fats from fatty fish, flaxseeds, and phospholipids are particularly important.

Boost your supply of acetylcholine. This neurotransmitter is key to improving memory and mental alertness—people suffering from Alzheimer's disease, for instance, show a marked deficiency in acetylcholine. Happily, it's easy to do this by taking choline and DMAE, two supplements that we'll discuss later in this chapter. It's vital to remember, however, that while acetylcholine is a major player as far as memory is concerned, it is only one of many in a large cast of neurotransmitters. Some stimulate mental processes, while others calm down information overload. You need the right balance.

It can help to look at the family tree of the neurotransmitter GABA and its cousins, glutamate and glutamine (see Figure 1 on page 24). The stimulating neurotransmitter glutamate helps to forge links between memories. This is how the taste enhancer MSG (monosodium glutamate), notoriously used in many Chinese restaurants, turns up the volume on tastes. But too much of it can definitely be a bad thing. GABA, a close relative of glutamate, calms the nervous system. If you want to enjoy good memory throughout your life, you have to get the right balance of these neurotransmitters.

And there's more—a range of substances that can give our minds and memories that extra boost. First, we'll take a brief look below at what's available from the pharmaceuticals companies. Then, we'll see how we can truly master our minds once again with natural alternatives.

SMART DRUGS AND HORMONES: A SELECT FEW

With age-related loss of memory on the increase and a growing demand for better mental performance to fit our multitasking lifestyles, it's no surprise that a new family of mind boosters has burst on the scene—the smart drugs. Although prescribed for people with diagnosed memory problems, they have a growing underground following.

More than 100 smart drugs, or *nootropics,* have emerged recently. The word, pronounced "no-a-tropic," means that they "enhance cognition." Some nootropics block the breakdown of neurotransmitters. Others mimic or improve the action of neurotransmitters, and still others are manufactured versions of hormones that influence brain function. Though an interesting lot, we don't discuss them here since they are available by prescription only, and some are not even readily available in the United States. (For more details, see the feature on smart drugs and hormones on www.naturalhighsbook.com and www.ceri.org.) Besides, there are enough natural, easily obtainable alternatives that are quite effective.

Natural Mind and Memory Boosters

If smart drugs are out, what about smart nutrients? There are several natural mind and memory boosters that can restore your clarity of thought and banish memory lapses. They are:

- Choline and DMAE—building blocks of acetylcholine.
- Pyroglutamate, phosphatidylserine, and omega-3 fats—receptor enhancers.
- Ginkgo (*ginkgo biloba*) and vinpocetine—circulation improvers.
- Acetyl-L-carnitine and glutamine—fuel for brain cells.
- Specific supporting vitamins and minerals.

With the exception of ginkgo, these are all substances found in food and the brain. They're becoming widely available, and you can buy combination state-of-the-art brain-boosting supplements in health food stores. We'll look at each in turn, then discuss why combining smart nutrients works best.

CHOLINE: THE BUILDING BLOCK OF MEMORY

The key brain chemical for memory is acetylcholine. A deficiency in this chemical is probably the single most common cause for declining memory. Acetylcholine is derived from the nutrient choline. Fish, especially sardines, are rich in it, hence the old wives' tale of fish being good for the brain. Eggs are also a major source of choline, followed by liver, soy beans, peanuts, and other nuts. Ever since egg phobia set in, the average intake of choline from the diet has dropped dramatically. From the point of view of memory enhancement, it is certainly worth eating more eggs. But just eating choline-rich foods won't do it. You also need vitamins B_5 (pantothenic acid), B_1, B_{12}, and C to form acetylcholine in your body.

Supplementing choline has some truly remarkable effects. Recent research at Duke University Medical Center demonstrated that giving choline to pregnant female rats created the equivalent of "superbrains" in the offspring. The researchers fed pregnant rats choline halfway through their pregnancy. The infant rats of mothers who received choline had vastly superior brains with more neuronal connections and, consequently, improved learning ability and better memory recall, all of which persisted into old age. This research showed that giving choline helps restructure the brain for improved performance. Based on this and numerous other studies that support the brain-enhancing properties of choline, and the fact that choline has no known toxicity, supplementing with choline during pregnancy is likely to enhance an infant's brain development.

High doses of choline has also been proven to boost memory in adults. For example, Florence Safford of Florida International University gave forty-one people, ages fifty to eighty, 500 mg doses of choline every day for five weeks. The subjects reported having only *half* the number of incidents of memory lapses—such as forgetting names or losing things—as before. If you combine choline with other smart nutrients, such as pyroglutamate, you can achieve the same memory-boosting effect at lower doses.

In addition to making the memory neurotransmitter, acetylcholine, choline is also a vital raw material for building nerve cells and receptor sites for neurotransmitters. According to Massachusetts Institute of Technology's Dr. Richard Wurtman, piracetam and other nootropic drugs that stimulate the release of acetylcholine should always be taken with choline. Otherwise, if choline levels are depleted, your body will divert the choline needed to build vital nerve cells into the production of more acetylcholine.

Some forms of choline cross more easily from the blood into the brain, referred to as "crossing the blood-brain barrier." These forms include phosphatidyl choline and a precursor for choline called DMAE (short for dimethylaminoethanol), which we'll investigate below. Phosphatidyl choline, or PC for short, is also found in lecithin, a supplement widely available in granules or capsules. Pure choline imparts a fishy smell, so you may prefer to use lecithin or PC.

A form of choline called citicholine has been used as a precursor to acetylcholine. It also boosts levels of dopamine and other neurotransmitters. It has even been used to treat victims of head injuries and strokes, since it protects brain cells from ischemia (decreased blood flow). It has also been shown to improve memory and learning in the elderly.

Recently a more potent form of choline, derived from soy lecithin, has become available in the United States. Alpha-GPC (L-alpha-glyceryl-phosphorylcholine, or choline alfoscerate) has a long history of use in Europe. Research on more than 3,000 patients and volunteers has shown Alpha-GPC to be more effective than citicholine, and with very few side effects (fifteen reported cases of diarrhea, dizziness, insomnia, or restlessness that resolved when the product was stopped). Besides possessing all the positive effects of citicholine, Alpha-GPC has also been shown to enhance the release of human growth hormone, the master antiaging hormone. Research with athletes has shown that it improves coordination, balance, and endurance. A limiting factor in its use has been its unavailability. However, we have discovered a source, which is listed in the Resources. Their Web site carries further product information (www.futurefoods.com). The recommended dose is 500–1,500 mg daily.

Choline

How it works: Precursor for the neurotransmitter acetylcholine; part of the structure of neuronal membranes.

Positive effects: More alert, clear-headed, better memory and concentration; improved brain development during gestation (pregnancy).

Cautions: None.

Dosage: 5–10 g (approximately 1 tablespoon) of lecithin, *or* 2.5–5 g (a heaping tablespoon) of hi-phosphatidylcholine lecithin, *or* 1–2 g of phosphatidyl choline, *or* 500 mg–2 g of choline chloride (fishy smelling); and 500–1,000 mg of citicholine and 500–1,500 mg of alpha-GPC. Take daily.

DMAE (DIMETHYLAMINOETHANOL): LET'S CONCENTRATE

DMAE, like choline, is plentiful in sardines and anchovies, but it crosses the blood-brain barrier and gets into the brain cells more rapidly. Once there, DMAE is a great natural mind and memory booster. DMAE accelerates the production of acetylcholine, reduces anxiety and racing minds, improves concentration and learning, and acts as a mild brain stimulant.

The ability of DMAE to tune up your brain was well demonstrated in a German study from 1996 with a group of adults with cognitive problems. The participants had their brain waves measured by an electroencephalogram (EEG) and were then given either DMAE or a placebo. There were no EEG changes measured in those taking the placebo, but those taking DMAE showed EEG improvements in brain-wave patterns in parts of the brain that play an important role in memory, attention, and flexibility of thinking.

A variation of DMAE is marketed as the drugs Deaner and Deanol. Numerous studies have shown that these drugs help people with learning problems, attention deficit disorder (ADD), and memory and behavioral problems. In one survey by Dr. Bernard Rimland from the Autism Research Institute in San Diego, Deaner was found to be almost twice as effective in treating children with ADD than the widely used drug Ritalin, without the side effects.

After thoroughly investigating the actions of DMAE, researcher and psychiatrist Charles Gant discovered that, in addition to increasing acetylcholine, DMAE in higher doses can actually block the acetylcholine receptor. This allows more dopamine to be released, thereby stimulating the brain as well. This action explains DMAE's success with reward deficiency syndrome and ADD.

If you want to boost your memory, the ideal dose of DMAE is 100–300 mg daily, taken in the morning or midday, not in the evening. Don't expect immediate results: DMAE can take two to three weeks to work. But it's worth waiting for.

Here's what three people shared about their experiences:

I've been taking DMAE for several weeks, and I've noticed an amazing difference in mood and concentration level.

AFB, AUSTIN, TEXAS

I am currently taking 100 mg of DMAE per day and notice a real difference in my alertness, energy level, and decreased need for sleep.

RS, SEATTLE, WASHINGTON

I've been using DMAE with pantothenic acid and a good multivitamin for two months now. One of the first things I noticed was that I fall asleep faster and wake up with a clearer mind. I experience a much sounder, more restful sleep. I constantly feel more attuned to my creative potential, and I'm always in a good mood. I truly feel alive and awake.

PW, NEW YORK, NEW YORK

DMAE

How it works: Precursor for choline that crosses readily into the brain, thereby helping to make acetylcholine. In higher doses, may act as a stimulant by enhancing dopamine activity.

Positive effects: Increases alertness; improves concentration; reduces anxiety; improves learning and attention span; normalizes brain-wave patterns.

Cautions: Too much can overstimulate and is therefore not recommended for those diagnosed with schizophrenia, mania, or epilepsy. Lower the dosage if you experience insomnia.

Dosage: 100–300 mg daily, taken in the morning or midday, not in the evening.

PYROGLUTAMATE, PHOSPHATIDYLSERINE, AND OMEGA-3 FATTY ACIDS: GET RECEPTIVE

The ability of neurotransmitters to deliver their message depends on having fully functioning receptor sites. These receptor sites need two key nutrients—phosphatidylserine (PS) and the omega-3 fat DHA. The amino acid pyroglutamate also has been found to vastly improve the brain's ability to receive messages, which in turn promotes learning and memory by increasing the number of acetylcholine receptor sites and improving their reception.

Pyroglutamate: The Master of Communication

Highly concentrated in the brain and spinal fluid, pyroglutamate is a key amino acid for enhancing memory and mental function. So powerful are its effects that many variations are now being marketed as nootropic drugs for learning and memory-related problems such as Alzheimer's disease. Numerous studies using these drugs, such as piracetam, have proven that they enhance memory and mental function, not only in people with pronounced memory decline but also in those with so-called "normal" memory function.

Pyroglutamate does the following three things that help improve memory and mental alertness:

- Increases acetylcholine production.
- Boosts the number of receptors for acetylcholine.
- Improves communication between the left and right hemispheres of the brain.

Pyroglutamate

How it works: Increases acetylcholine production; improves reception.

Positive effects: Improves memory, cognitive function, concentration, coordination, and reaction time; improves communication between the right and left hemispheres of the brain.

Cautions: None.

Dosage: 300–1,000 mg a day.

In other words, pyroglutamate improves the brain's internal talking, listening, and cooperation. This is likely how it improves learning, memory, concentration, and the speed of reflexes. It can really give you an extra mental edge.

Pyroglutamate is found in many foods, including fish, dairy products, fruit, and vegetables. Arginine pyroglutamate is one of its more common forms used in brain-boosting supplements.

Phosphatidylserine: The Memory Molecule

Known as "the memory molecule," phosphatidylserine (PS) can genuinely give some oomph to the brain. A member of the family of phospholipids, discussed in Chapter 3, it is essential for the health of the liver, immune system, nerves, and brain. It is especially plentiful in the brain, and there's increasing evidence that supplementing with it can improve memory, mood, stress resistance, learning, and concentration. The secret to the memory-boosting properties of PS is probably due to its ability to help brain cells communicate. This is because PS is the main component of the "docking port" for neurotransmitters such as acetylcholine.

While the body can make its own PS, we still rely on receiving some directly from diet, which makes it a semi-essential nutrient. The trouble is

Phosphatidylserine

How it works: Building material for neuronal membranes and neurotransmitter receptor sites.

Positive effects: Improves mood, memory, stress resistance, learning, and concentration.

Cautions: None.

Dosage: 100–300 mg a day.

that modern diets are deficient in PS unless you happen to eat a lot of organ meats, which can supply about 50 mg a day. A typical vegetarian diet is unlikely to provide even 10 mg a day, so a supplement is usually needed.

PS is particularly helpful for people with learning difficulties or age-related memory decline. In one study, supplementing with PS improved the subjects' memories to the level of people twelve years younger. Dr. Thomas Crook from the Memory Assessment Clinic in Bethesda, Maryland, gave 149 people with age-associated memory impairment a daily dose of 300 mg of PS or a placebo. When tested after twelve weeks, the ability of those taking PS to match names to faces (a recognized measure of memory and mental function) vastly improved.

Omega-3 Fats: Why Fish Is Good for the Brain

As your grandmother may have told you, fish is good for the brain. But she may not have understood that the mind-boosting powers of fish such as salmon, tuna, and mackerel are derived from the essential fats they contain. As we've already seen, EPA and DHA, found mainly in fatty fish and also in flaxseed, hemp, and walnut oils, are omega-3 fats that uniquely feed the brain. (See Chapter 3.)

DHA, more than EPA, is highly concentrated in our brains and nervous systems, and improves not only learning and age-related memory but also mood. The higher your blood levels of DHA, the higher your levels of acetylcholine and serotonin are likely to be. The reason for this is that DHA builds receptor sites and improves reception. According to Dr. J. R. Hibbeln, who noticed that fish eaters are less prone to depression, "It's like building more serotonin factories, instead of just increasing the efficiency of the serotonin you have."

In one study, when people with bipolar or manic depression were given 9.6 mg of omega-3 oils over a four-month period, they experienced substantial improvement. DHA has also been found to improve dyslexia (difficulty reading) and dyspraxia (clumsiness). Dr. Jaqueline Stordy of the University of Surrey found that DHA improves the reading ability and behavior of adults with dyslexia.

EPA is proving to be the more important omega-3 fat for treating schizophrenia. While not directly involved in building the receptor sites, EPA makes prostaglandins—unique information molecules that also tune up the brain and promote healthy brain function. So EPA is a fat that is more involved in the transmission of information, while DHA is more involved in the reception, which is why we need both.

An ideal intake of EPA and DHA is in the order of 500–1,000 mg a day, or double if you have one of the mental health problems we've discussed above. Most fish oils provide about equal amounts of EPA and DHA, so your actual DHA requirement is half this—250–500 mg. Alternatively, you can eat a 3-ounce serving of fish, preferably mackerel, herring, sardines, tuna, or salmon, three times a week.

The most concentrated supplements provide 700 mg per capsule. A good-quality cod liver oil supplement can provide up to 400 mg of EPA and DHA in total but should not be taken in higher doses because of its high vitamin A content. (While important, this fat-soluble vitamin should not be taken in excess.) For vegetarians, flaxseed oil is the most direct source of omega-3 fats. You need the equivalent of either a level tablespoon of flaxseeds or a tablespoon of flaxseed oil, also available in capsules. Since each capsule usually provides 1,000 mg of the oil, you will need eight of these to get the equivalent of a tablespoon of flaxseed oil. Or use algae-based DHA capsules.

Since these fragile oils are subject to oxidation, both in the bottle and in your brain, you need to accompany this with the antioxidant and fat-soluble vitamin E, 400–800 IU daily.

Best Fish for Brain Fats (Amount of DHA in a 3-ounce Serving)	
Mackerel	1,400 mg
Herring	1,000 mg
Sardines	1,000 mg
Tuna	900 mg
Anchovy	900 mg
Salmon	800 mg
Trout	500 mg

EPA

How it works: Precursor for prostaglandins, chemicals that influence mood and behavior and probably affect neurotransmitter balance.

Positive effects: Helps restore normal mood in bipolar illness; may also affect memory.

Cautions: EPA helps reduce blood clotting; therefore, high doses should not be taken if you are on blood-thinning medication.

Dosage: 250–1,000 mg a day as a fish oil supplement, or eat 3 ounces of fatty fish three times a week. Take with 400–800 IU of vitamin E daily.

DHA

How it works: Building material for neuronal membranes and neurotransmitter receptor sites; increases acetylcholine and serotonin levels.

Positive effects: Improves learning, memory, and mood in depression, manic depression, dyslexia, and dyspraxia.

Cautions: DHA helps reduce blood clotting; therefore, high doses should not be taken if you are on blood-thinning medication.

Dosage: 250–1,000 mg a day as a fish oil supplement, or eat 3 ounces of fatty fish three times a week. Algae-based products are also available (e.g., Neuromins by Martek).

The omega-6 fatty acids, GLA (gamma-linolenic acid) and LA (linoleic acid), are also important for brain function. The recommended ratio of the omega-6 to omega-3 is 1:1. The former are abundant in our diets, in vegetable oils, meats, and dairy products, producing a ratio of 20:1 or 30:1, in favor of omega-6 oils. Thus, we generally have a relative deficiency in omega-3 over omega-6 oils. Nonetheless, when necessary to supplement, we recommend evening primrose oil, borage oil, pumpkin oil, or hemp oil, supplying 1,000 mg daily.

GINKGO BILOBA: ENHANCE YOUR CIRCULATION

Ginkgo (*Ginkgo biloba*) is an herbal remedy for memory enhancement that has been used in the East for thousands of years. Coming from one of the oldest known species of trees, the first medicinal uses of ginkgo can be traced back to 2800 B.C. Research has shown that ginkgo improves short-term and age-related memory loss, slow thinking, depression, circulation, and poor blood flow to the brain. It has also been seen to significantly improve both Parkinson's and Alzheimer's diseases over the course of a year. Ginkgo's remarkable healing properties appear to come from two constituent chemicals—flavonoids and terpene lactones.

As well as being a powerful antioxidant that helps vitamin E and other antioxidant nutrients protect the brain from damage, ginkgo also aids in the production of neurotransmitters and helps to normalize acetylcholine receptors. However, its major benefit is its ability to improve the circulation of blood within the brain by mildly dilating blood vessels and inhibiting the action of platelet-activating factor, a substance that thickens the blood. So, ultimately, ginkgo helps to get oxygen and other important nutrients into the brain.

A review of forty studies testing ginkgo's effects on people with cerebral circulation problems, carried out by Jos Kleijnen and Paul Knipschild from the University of Limburg in the Netherlands, found significant improvement in memory, concentration, energy, and mood. After isolating the eight trials that met the highest methodological standards, they found that 70 percent of those receiving ginkgo (120–160 mg daily for twelve weeks) showed improvement, compared with 14 percent of those receiving a placebo.

A comprehensive double-blind placebo-controlled trial involving 309 Alzheimer's disease outpatients, ages sixty to eighty, was published by P. L. Le Bars and colleagues in the prestigious *Journal of the American Medical Association*. In the 212 subjects who completed the year-long study, there was significant improvement in cognition and social performance.

Ginseng seems to fire the action of ginkgo. A recent experiment carried out by Professor Keith Wesnes at the University of Northumbria gave 256 healthy volunteers between the ages of thirty-six and sixty-six either a combination of ginkgo and ginseng or a placebo. After fourteen weeks, people taking the herbal combination performed much better in memory tests. According to one volunteer, "I felt like I was thinking clearer and wasn't so mentally drained at the end of a long stressful day. I noticed I was able to recall things that I had trouble remembering before."

Ginkgo is usually taken in capsule form, standardized at a flavonoid concentration of 24 percent. It may come in capsules of 40 mg, 60 mg, 80 mg, and 120 mg, with 60 mg the most common. The recommended dose range is 120–180 mg of extract daily, which is one to two of the 60-mg capsules twice a day. It often takes a month or two of consistent use before

Ginkgo Biloba

How it works: Improves circulation; acts as an antioxidant.

Positive effects: Improves mood, memory, concentration, and energy.

Cautions: Use with caution if taking blood-thinning medication. Rare side effects of headaches, nausea, or nosebleeds have been reported at high doses.

Dosage: 120–240 mg a day of a standardized extract providing 24 percent flavonoids, taken in two doses a day (60–120 mg twice daily).

you begin to see results. If you see none after eight to ten weeks, you can then increase the dose to 240 mg—two capsules of 60 mg twice daily.

Ginkgo is a blood-thinning agent, so you must use caution if you're taking other blood thinners such as coumadin, heparin, or even aspirin. Side effects such as headaches, nausea, or nosebleeds have been reported, but only rarely and at higher doses.

VINPOCETINE: THE SECRET OF THE PERIWINKLE

Vinpocetine, the active ingredient of the periwinkle plant (*Vinca minor*), has been available as a cognitive enhancer since 1998. Like ginkgo, vinpocetine improves blood flow and circulation, thus helping deliver oxygen to the brain. There have been many studies to support its efficacy, including one at the University of Surrey in Guildford, England. In this double-blind placebo-controlled study, researchers gave 203 people with memory problems either a placebo or 10–20 mg of vinpocetine. Those on the vinpocetine showed a significant improvement in cognitive performance, with a slight edge to the higher dose group. Research in Russia has also found vinpocetine to be potentially helpful for those with epilepsy.

According to a seventy-two-year-old man with ARCD, "I take a 5-mg

Vinpocetine

How it works: Improves blood flow and circulation to the brain.

Positive effects: Improves cognitive performance; potentially helpful in epilepsy.

Cautions: None reported.

Dosage: 10–40 mg a day. Increase dosage gradually but do not exceed 40 mg daily.

dose of vinpocetine at breakfast and lunch. I feel more focused, and it seems that I can make decisions quicker. I also notice colors to be more vivid."

Vinpocetine is available in 5-mg and 10-mg pills. Peak blood levels occur one and a half hours after ingestion. It is best to start with 5 mg twice daily, and build up slowly. Although there are no known adverse effects, we have no long-term studies at high doses, so it's best to be cautious in raising the dose.

ACETYL-L-CARNITINE: THE BRAIN'S SUPERFUEL

The amino acid carnitine can be used directly as brain fuel. Acetyl-L-carnitine (ALC) is especially useful because the "acetyl" part helps to make acetylcholine, the key memory neurotransmitter. Supplementing ALC helps to promote both acetylcholine production and release.

ALC also acts as an antioxidant that protects against brain damage and keeps your nervous system youthful. In animals, ALC helps to stimulate the growth of new brain cells and improve communication between the right and left hemispheres of the brain.

Acetyl-L-carnitine (ALC)

How it works: Fuel for the brain; helps make acetylcholine; acts as an antioxidant.

Positive effects: Improves mood and mental performance.

Cautions: Not recommended for those with diabetes, liver disease, or kidney disease.

Dosage: 250–1,500 mg daily, between meals.

Plenty of studies have proven ALC's mind- and mood-enhancing prop-erties. You need between 250 and 1,500 mg for a noticeable effect. ALC be-comes even more effective if taken with phosphatidylserine. Unfortunately, it is very expensive and is perhaps not a smart nutrient of choice for this reason. It's best to take it some time before or after eating for maximum absorption.

GLUTAMINE: MORE SUPERFUEL

Glutamine, another amino acid, is also used directly as fuel for the brain. Glutamine has been shown to both enhance mental performance and to de-crease addictive tendencies. Supplementing glutamine, which the brain uses to build and balance the neurotransmitters GABA and glutamate, can help promote memory. It can be a very useful addition to a supplement pro-gram if you are breaking your addiction to sugar or stimulants (see Chapter 5). We recommend 2–5 g a day, the equivalent of a teaspoon of glutamine powder, which is much more cost effective than tablets. It is best taken be-tween meals for maximum absorption.

Glutamine

How it works: Fuel for brain cells; helps build and balance neurotrans-mitters.

Positive effects: Improves both mental energy and relaxation; reduces addiction; stabilizes blood sugar; promotes memory.

Cautions: Rare reports of headaches at high doses.

Dosage: 2–5 g a day, between meals, for maximum absorption.

VITAMINS AND MINERALS: A BRAIN'S BEST FRIEND

It's official: multivitamins and minerals make you brainier. This was first proven by a research study involving ninety students, carried out by Gwilym Roberts, a schoolteacher and nutritionist from the Institute for Optimum Nutrition, and Dr. David Benton, a psychologist from the Department of Psychology at Swansea University College in Wales. Sixty students were given either a special multivitamin and mineral supplement designed to ensure an optimal intake of key nutrients or a placebo. Thirty students, serving as a control group, were given no supplement at all. After eight months, the IQs of those taking the supplements had risen by over ten points! No changes were seen in those taking the placebos, or in the control group.

More than a dozen similar studies have been done since and, even with smaller nutrient doses, lower but still significant IQ changes have been reported. For example, a study at the University of California revealed an average increase of 4.4 IQ points in students receiving only the recommended dietary allowance (RDA) level of vitamins and minerals. Almost half of the students on supplements had an increase in IQ of fifteen or more points.

Exactly how vitamin and mineral supplementation increases IQ scores was discovered by psychologist Wendy Snowden from Reading University's Department of Psychology. In her trial, she also gave children either supplements or placebos. Those children receiving the supplements showed significant increases in IQ scores after ten weeks. A close analysis of performance in the IQ tests showed the same error rate, but fewer unanswered questions after the ten weeks of supplementation. Since almost all the unanswered questions came toward the end of the test, when the children ran out of time, the children on supplements seemed to answer questions faster (hence fewer omissions). This suggests that the effect of the vitamin and mineral supplements was to increase the speed of processing, perhaps by increasing concentration, which is clearly a significant factor in intelligence. In other words, vitamins don't increase your inherent intelligence, but they *do* help you to think faster and concentrate longer.

While few similar studies have been performed on adults, it's highly likely that optimum intakes of vitamins and minerals can improve their concentration and speed of information processing as well. One study carried out by Dr. Benton at Swansea University College gave 127 adults ten times the RDA levels of vitamins and minerals, or dummy pills. After twelve months, the women were showing real improvement in attention and mental performance. Why the men didn't show similar improvements remains a mystery.

Of all the vitamins and minerals, B vitamins have the most important role in ensuring optimal brain function due to their vital role in delivering oxygen to the brain and protecting it from harmful free radicals. B vitamins also turn glucose into energy within the brain cells and assist in the manufacture of neurotransmitters. B vitamins are, in short, your brain's very best friends. Let's see how they do it.

• Vitamin B_3 (niacin) is particularly good at enhancing memory. In one study, subjects of various ages received 141 mg of niacin a day. Memory was improved by 10 to 40 percent in all age groups.

• Vitamin B_5 (pantothenic acid) helps improve memory and mental alertness. You can sharpen your memory by taking 250–500 mg a day. As you've learned, vitamin B_5 is essential for the formation of acetylcholine.

• Vitamin B_6 (pyridoxine) is necessary for making neurotransmitters. It's also necessary for converting amino acids into the important neurotransmitter serotonin—a deficiency of which can cause depression and other problems. One study found that about one-fifth of depressed people who participated were deficient in pyridoxine. Even 20 mg a day can improve memory, but suggested supplementation is 20–100 mg a day.

• Vitamin B_{12} (cyanocobalamin) has been shown in laboratory experiments to speed up the rate at which rats learn. Because B_{12} is essential for the health of nerve cells, its absence is a prime cause of mental deterioration and confusion in older people. A dosage of 10–100 mcg of B_{12} a day is usually sufficient. Older people often have very poor absorption of B_{12}, and may benefit from much higher amounts, such as 1,000 mcg daily. Taking B_{12} in an under-the-tongue formula improves its absorption.

• Folic acid, like vitamin B_{12}, is essential for oxygen delivery to the brain. A deficiency in either causes macrocytic or large cell anemia, meaning that the red blood cells actually enlarge in order to carry more oxygen, since they are short of these nutrients. You need about 400 mcg of folic acid daily.

B Vitamins

How they work: Turn glucose into energy in neurons; cofactors for making neurotransmitters; help transport oxygen; protect the brain from toxins and oxidants.

Positive effects: Raise IQ; improve energy, memory, mood, and concentration.

Cautions: None when taken in sensible doses. Excess B_3 and B_6 can have adverse effects, so don't exceed the recommended doses. B_3 as niacin acts as a vasodilator, improving circulation and causing flushing at doses above 50 mg.

Dosage: 50–500 mg daily of each of the following: B_1, B_2, B_3, and B_6; 50–500 mg of B_5; 10–1,000 mcg of B_{12}; 400–800 mcg of folic acid (daily).

SYNERGY: TOGETHER WE'RE TERRIFIC

Each of these proven mind boosters is remarkable in its own right, but together they can really rev up your brainpower. Supplementing smart nutrients, such as phosphatidyl choline, pantothenic acid, DMAE, and pyroglutamate, in combination boosts mind and memory far more than when taken individually. Consider the following study: A team of researchers led by Raymond Bartus gave choline and piracetam, a derivative of pyroglutamate, either separately or in combination to aged lab rats noted for their age-related memory decline. The team reported that the "rats given the piracetam/choline combination exhibited memory retention scores several times better than those with piracetam alone." A study on humans was then carried out by Dr. S. Ferris and associates at New York University School of Medicine. These researchers, too, found dramatic clinical improvements in subjects, way beyond those given either choline or piracetam separately.

While both choline and piracetam improved memory, the results showed that half the dose was needed with a choline/piracetam combo. This illustrates the power of combining just two smart nutrients. We recommend combining all the smart nutrients discussed in this chapter for the most effective natural mind and memory boost.

Some smart nutrient supplements contain combinations of all these acetylcholine-friendly nutrients—choline, DMAE, pantothenic acid, and pyroglutamate. The ideal doses are less when combined than when a substance is taken alone. If you want to shine mentally and fit names to faces with ease, take the smart nutrients listed in the following section, in the doses indicated.

ACTION PLAN TO BOOST MIND AND MEMORY

To hone your cognitive abilities and memory, you may need to make some changes in your diet supplementation. Here's a summary of our recommendations:

- Eat fish three times a week, with preference for mackerel, herring, sardines, tuna, or salmon. Vegetarians need to have a tablespoon of ground flaxseeds a day, or a tablespoon of flaxseed oil. Or take a EPA/DHA rich fish oil supplement.
- Supplement a good all-round multivitamin supplying optimal amounts of B vitamins.
- Supplement a "smart nutrient" formula providing the nutrients and amounts shown below. (See Supplement Directory on page 206.)
- Take a tablespoon of lecithin or a heaping teaspoon of hi-PC lecithin a day. (Smart nutrient formulas rarely contain enough phosphatidylcholine because it's bulky.)
- If you are over age fifty or if you are suffering from age-related memory decline, consider adding one or more of the following daily, in divided doses with food: 100–300 mg of phosphatidylserine; 500–1,000 mg of EPA/DHA; 500–5,000 mg (a heaping

teaspoon) of glutamine; 1,000 mg of acetyl-L-carnitine; and 500–1,500 mg of alpha-GPC.

For a full natural mind-enhancement program, see Top Tips in Part Four.

Smart Nutrients	Daily Dose
Phosphatidylcholine (PC)	200–2,000 mg
DMAE	200–400 mg
Pyroglutamate	300–1,000 mg
Phosphatidylserine (PS)	50–200 mg
EPA and DHA* combination	1,000 mg
Ginkgo Biloba	120–240 mg
Vinpocetine	10–40 mg
Vitamin B_3 (niacin)	40–200 mg
Vitamin B_5 (pantothenic acid)	200–500 mg
Vitamin B_6 (pyridoxine)	20–100 mg
Vitamin B_{12} (cyanocobalamin)	10–1,000 mcg
Folic acid	400–800 mcg

*DHA as an oil cannot be added to dry supplements. However, it is available in a more expensive powder form in some supplement combinations.

8

Making the Connection

If the doors of perception were cleansed everything
would appear to man as it is: Infinite.
WILLIAM BLAKE

The Need to Connect

It may hit you when you're with close friends, the person you love, or wandering alone in a beautiful place: that feeling of being at one with the world. Such experiences help to shape and motivate us, and leave us feeling joyful, at peace, and part of something bigger than us—in short, connected. Food, clothing, and shelter are survival basics, but feeling connected may be the most vital of all.

Of course there are other ways to connect, such as getting drunk or stoned with friends on a Saturday night. But, in this case, it's not only the company, it's also the chemicals and their inhibition-stripping actions that make us feel that sense of connection.

Some of us, sometimes, feel the need to connect far more strongly. We may be going through a bleak period or experiencing a sense of not belonging. Or we may be searching for meaning and for spiritual connection. All this can lead to experimenting with "love drugs" such as Ecstasy or psychedelics such as LSD. Sometimes it's peer pressure—"all my friends are doing it"—that makes it happen.

These psychoactive substances, though, have their downsides. Fortunately, we have found that there are certain natural herbs and nutrients that can help you feel part of it all, not apart. You'll find ways of blissing out and opening up your mind to new frontiers by using these natural substances to access your brain's own pharmacopia.

THE CHEMISTRY OF CONNECTION

Feeling good about yourself and connected to others has a lot to do with your mental and spiritual health. But, as we know, it also gets down to chemistry. Besides the drama of trauma, we've seen how a lack of GABA makes you feel stressed, a lack of dopamine makes you unmotivated, a deficiency of serotonin leaves you depressed, and insufficient acetylcholine leads to mental exhaustion. A big part of feeling connected is having all of these neurotransmitters in proper balance so that you are firing on all cylinders.

So, the best opening strategy for feeling connected and happy is to learn how to fine-tune your brain through diet, supplements, and lifestyle changes, as we've outlined so far. The resulting sense of energy and well-being is the perfect springboard for higher experiences.

PEAK EXPERIENCES: THE BIGGER PICTURE

We all seek happiness, confidence, security, and self-esteem. Once these things are achieved, some of us may even feel complacent. But then there is a deeper human urge—to discover life's meaning and purpose. This urge may spark a quest for transcendent or "peak" experiences in which you have a greater sense of unity or harmony, within yourself, with others, and with life itself. These are the flashes of inspiration that often fuel great works of music, art, and poetry, as well as scientific and spiritual breakthroughs.

By their very nature, peak experiences are difficult to put into words. Patrick remembers having such an experience while meditating:

The meaning in life is the slightest shift like driving a car round the corner into a panoramic view or breaking through fathoms of dim water into the light. Nothing is different; nothing is the same. What once was your life is now only a game. Like breathing air for the very first time, it feels so natural; it feels so right to be bathing in this radiant light.

The experience gave Patrick a whole new perspective on various problems that he was grappling with at the time.

Many of us have been fortunate enough to have had similar peak experiences. Perhaps you were deeply in love, or had a profound, life-changing insight. You may have caught a flash of the "bigger picture," or of the connectedness of everything, when you were in the midst of stunning natural beauty. You may have experienced a spiritual awakening through meditation or another discipline, or had a drug-induced, mind-altering experience.

Highly traumatic, life-threatening events and near-death experiences are some of the fastest ways to achieve peak or transcendent states of mind. Such events put our minds and bodies into emergency mode and cause the release of a slew of brain chemicals that may be nature's way of protecting us, at least temporarily, from a scary reality. Many report these experiences as life-changing. What had seemed important becomes trivial when faced with life or death. There may be a resulting spiritual transformation that leads to an urge to share, to comfort, and to serve others, and, in some way, "to report from the front lines." For details, see books by Kenneth Ring and others on near-death experiences. Most of us haven't had—nor wish to have—this high drama as a path to enlightenment.

Others have used psychoactive drugs known as *entheogens*—substances that awaken or generate mystical experiences. Literally meaning "toward god," these substances include Ecstasy (MDMA), psilocybin mushrooms, and LSD. Take Jerome's experience, for example. This seventy-year-old retired engineer took pure MDMA (Ecstasy), legally in 1980, under the guidance of a psychotherapist:

Before, I had thought of reality as being just the concrete reality that we see before us. MDMA made me see other, generally invisible realities, almost visions, that coexist with it. I could see the intercon-

nectedness of all people and all things, and felt a powerful love ema-
nating from within me. I saw my partner in a totally different way—
with absolute acceptance and love. It was an exquisite dance of
harmony and pure love. I became a happier, more fulfilled person,
more complete in many ways. It has colored my life ever since.

It's really not surprising that young people, separating from their first source of connection—their families—have embraced Ecstasy. In the U.S., an estimated 1 million Ecstasy tablets are taken every week, mainly by sixteen- to twenty-five-year-olds. Figures also show that use of such substances usually diminishes or stops as we age.

Without condoning the use of MDMA, which has many downsides (see page 170), the fact that a chemical can help to induce a life-changing, transcendent experience under certain circumstances warrants investigation. In our search for natural highs, we want to know what's going on in the brain during peak experiences, whether chemically induced or not, and discover natural ways to bliss-out without the downsides. In the following section, we'll be looking at forty years of research into the chemistry of connection. The study of how entheogens alter consciousness has led to discoveries that can open doors to a natural high. But first, let's cover some background.

PLATO TOOK ACID: THE HISTORY OF GETTING HIGH

In case you think the use of entheogens has little relevance to humanity's quest for getting high, take a look at history. Virtually every culture throughout history has used these substances. In India almost 4,000 years ago, the Vedas—ancient Hindu philosophical texts—extolled a plant potion called *soma*, considered to be God in plant form. The ancient Greeks, from Aristotle to Plato, took part in an initiation ceremony called the Eleusian mysteries that involved consuming a rye-based drink. Historians believe this contained the ergot-rye fungus, a natural source of LSD. Egyptian cultures used the blue lily, henbane, and mandrake, which were also favorites of European witches.

In the Americas, the Mayans discovered that certain mushrooms and the skin of certain toads contained powerful hallucinogens. Some Native American tribes still use the peyote cactus to this day. Probably the earliest use of "magic" mushrooms predates even this, back to the Siberian peoples of northeast Asia, who later crossed the Bering Strait to colonize the Americas. They revered the highly toxic *Amanita muscaria,* or fly agaric, a red-and-white spotted mushroom that Alice took to enter Wonderland in Lewis Carroll's classic story. To this day, an herbal brew known as *yage* or *ayahuasca* is still used widely by South American shamans.

In the West, the mostly widely used entheogens are "designer drugs," manufactured compounds such as Ecstasy (MDMA) and LSD.

EXPAND YOUR MIND: HOW ENTHEOGENS WORK

Our brains filter out the vast majority of information that comes in through our senses. This allows us to scan a mere fraction of what is actually out there and helps us to organize our world. We see only what we need to see for our survival.

When you take an entheogen, this filter is suspended, and you begin to see the bigger picture. It sounds amazing, and as we've seen in Jerome's story, it is. But there are some downsides to entheogens: the experiences aren't always good, and many have adverse side effects. We'll go into these below, but first let's see precisely how entheogens dissolve the filters in our brains. This will give us some vital clues to finding the best natural connectors.

DMT: Key to Connection

In the vast majority of entheogens, the active compounds are substances called tryptamines, related to tryptophan and serotonin (5-hydroxytryptamine). (See Figure 5.) The most active one is DMT (N,N-dimethyltryptamine), a tryptamine with two methyl groups, which is closely related to the "happy" neurotransmitter serotonin. DMT is thought to be primarily produced—along with serotonin and melatonin—in the pineal gland. DMT acts much like a neurotransmitter and is a mind-expanding substance in its own right.

The pineal gland, which is at the center of the brain, is light sensitive in many animals. It acts as a vital connection to their environment, perceiving

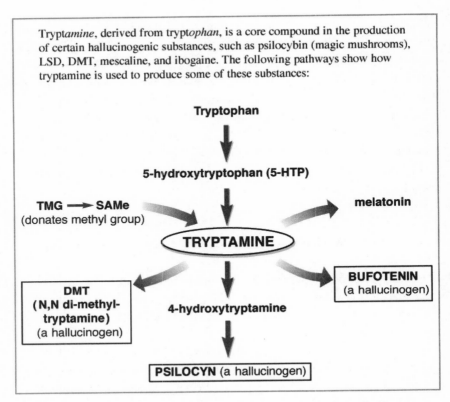

Tryptamine, derived from tryptophan, is a core compound in the production of certain hallucinogenic substances, such as psilocybin (magic mushrooms), LSD, DMT, mescaline, and ibogaine. The following pathways show how tryptamine is used to produce some of these substances:

Tryptophan

5-hydroxytryptophan (5-HTP)

TMG ⟶ SAMe
(donates methyl group)

melatonin

TRYPTAMINE

DMT
(N,N di-methyl-
tryptamine)
(a hallucinogen)

4-hydroxytryptamine

BUFOTENIN
(a hallucinogen)

PSILOCYN (a hallucinogen)

Figure 5. These pathways show how tryptamine is used to produce certain hallucinogenic substances.

the ebb and flow of day and night, as well as seasonal changes. The Indian mystics consider it our "third eye," an antenna for "inner light." Philosophers, including René Descartes, considered the pineal gland to be "the seat of the soul."

All entheogens have profound effects on the neurotransmitter serotonin and, perhaps most important, on DMT.

With DMT there is no tolerance or downregulation. Just like the neurotransmitters dopamine, serotonin, and acetylcholine, DMT works every time. This suggests that we all have within us the chemistry that is associated with expanded awareness and feeling connected, *all the time.*

Of course, most of us *don't* feel permanently connected. *Why not?* Perhaps it's partly because we don't make enough DMT, or our brains rapidly break down what little DMT we produce. At the University of New Mexico's School of Medicine, Dr. Rick Strassman discovered that DMT injected into the bloodstream produces an immediate change in consciousness. However, its effect only lasts about 15 to 30 minutes. For a fascinating exploration of DMT and its effects on conciousness, read Dr. Strassman's excellent book *DMT: The Spirit Molecule*.

While we have a long way to go in uncovering the chemistry of consciousness, it appears that neurotransmitter activity is involved in the action of our brains' selective filters. When these filters are suspended, we hear the whole symphony of life.

But how much exposure to infinity can we stand? Are mind-altering experiences always positive or desired? And, if so, are there downsides to the use of entheogens such as Ecstasy or LSD? And are there natural connectors, with no downsides? These are the questions we will explore in this chapter.

Magic Mushrooms, LSD, and Ecstasy: What Goes Up . . .

There are hundreds of natural entheogens, as well as a vast array of designer drugs, that are beyond the scope of this book. (For further reading, see Recommended Reading.) Let's just look at the most commonly used—psilocybin or "magic" mushrooms, LSD, and Ecstasy (MDMA). We'll start by looking at their downsides, beginning with the ones common to all entheogens.

Most entheogens have some level of tolerance and have some day-after depression (letdown). Depending on circumstances, there may be a strong pull to use the drug again, especially Ecstasy.

Since few people are likely to want to use hallucinogens (LSD or mushrooms) with any frequency, the greatest risk is a bad trip. In the face of the serious shock to your normal reality brought on by these substances, and without the appropriate preparation and support, you can become extremely anxious and fearful. If you are at all unstable, an experience like this could leave you quite emotionally fragile.

"Set," or expectation, and "setting," or environment, are of prime importance in how a psychedelic journey unfolds, as we have seen in traditional cultures or in therapeutic settings. A loud, crowded party may not be the place to trip. Think twice before taking an entheogen "just for fun." Far from experiencing a sense of connection, you may end up feeling extremely alienated from your own sense of being, as well as from other people.

PSILOCYBIN MUSHROOMS: HOW MAGIC ARE THEY?

Psilocybin is the major psychoactive agent in so-called "magic" mushrooms (*Psilocybe cubensis*). This is one of many tryptamine-containing fungi that have been used for thousands of years throughout Europe, Asia, and the Americas.

Depending on dosage, the effects of taking psilocybin mushrooms include greater emotional sensitivity, visual hallucinations, time distortion, nausea, and nervousness.

As with most entheogens, when the effects wear off, there is often a feeling of fogginess and fatigue, though sleep may not come easily. Occasionally, although the mushrooms are not toxic, very high doses can cause vomiting. Other species of psychoactive mushrooms, such as *Amanita muscaria* or fly agaric, can be toxic and even fatal.

LSD: THE ACID TEST

Lysergic acid diethylamide, abbreviated to LSD, was discovered in 1946 by Albert Hofmann while working for the Sandoz Pharmaceutical Company. In the 1960s and 1970s, popularized by Dr. Timothy Leary, it became the drug of choice of the counterculture. His research with LSD while a professor of psychology at Harvard inspired his famous exhortation to "turn on, tune in, and drop out"—and many did, including Leary himself. There are a number of excellent books that describe this era, its drugs, and its gurus. (See Recommended Reading.)

LSD, one of the most powerful entheogens, is produced from ergota-mine, which is found in fungi that typically grow on rye. A related com-pound, ergonovine, is found in several species of morning glory seeds. The amount needed to produce an effect is tiny compared to other entheogens (100 *micro*grams of LSD versus 100 *milli*grams of MDMA for a reasonable mind-altering experience—a factor of 1,000; that is, the effective dose of MDMA is 1,000 times that of LSD!).

LSD was used extensively in psychotherapy during the 1960s, with some benefit. An LSD experience is called a "trip" because it is much like a journey to another place. And, as we've indicated, this can be a very self-confrontational experience. Pioneering psychiatrist Oscar Janiger researched LSD in the 1950s and interviewed hundreds of people after LSD trips; he came to the following conclusion:

> *LSD seems to produce a marked shift in our fundamental percep-tual frame of reference, upon which rests our ongoing concept of real-ity. This change in our habitual way of being in the world may lead to a profound psychic shake-up and may provide startling insights into the nature of reality and into how our personal existence is fashioned.*

LSD should not be taken by anyone who is unstable or immature, is too strongly attached to his or her ego, has a preexisting, deep-seated emotional trauma, or suffers from mental illness.

LSD's other risk is that of its notorious "flashbacks." They are due to the imprinting in our memories, while under the influence, of powerful negative experiences. When triggered later, the initial experience may be re-experienced. This is similar to the posttraumatic stress disorder (PTSD) of war veterans, who may vividly recall a mortar attack after hearing a car backfire.

Despite its status as an illegal drug, LSD isn't actually physiologically addictive nor has it been found to damage the brain. Like other trypta-mines, it promotes the release of serotonin, followed by serotonin depletion. This can interfere with sleep that same night, making you feel tired and sub-dued the next day. Perhaps because the dose needed is so small, LSD is rela-tively nontoxic, and it has no known lethal dose. Any deaths related to LSD have been due to dangerous behavior secondary to its impairing the person's judgment, rather than to the drug itself. Some individuals taking LSD while under the supervision of a psychiatrist *in a therapeutic setting* have had psychological breakthroughs. However, LSD is now classified as a Schedule I drug, illegal except for use in research and with a special license.

LSD effects may include the following:

- Feelings of connection.
- Visual hallucinations.
- Time distortion.
- Increased sensory awareness—hypersensitivity to music, noise, and other stimuli.
- Synesthesia, a sensation where sounds are "seen" and visual stimuli are "heard."

In addition to the above, the following unwanted negative effects may also occur:

- Paranoia.
- Fear and panic.
- Overwhelming negative feelings.
- Flashbacks.
- Jaw tension.
- Sweating.
- Nausea.
- Dizziness.
- Impaired coordination and judgment.

THE AGONY OVER ECSTASY (MDMA)

Can It Be Deadly?

Deaths from Ecstasy use, even among first-time users, have been reported in the media. According to a thorough evaluation by the British Police Foundation: "Although deaths from Ecstasy are highly publicized, it probably kills fewer than ten people each year, which, though deeply distressing for the surviving relatives and friends, is a small percentage of the many thousands of people who use it each week." It's not really clear, though, exactly what killed these unfortunate few. Was it the MDMA itself or the cocktail of drugs in the pill sold as Ecstasy? Was it overheating from dancing all night, dehydration, or drinking too much water? It was certainly some combination of these, with many questions still to be answered by the appropriate research.

Can It Cause Brain Damage?

A real danger with Ecstasy appears to be that of young people buying so-called Ecstasy at raves (large dance parties). They may be getting a cocktail of amphetamine and other stimulants or hallucinogens, with perhaps no MDMA in it at all. An organization called Dance Safe (www.dancesafe.org) has volunteered at raves to analyze the products sold. This, too, has become a controversial practice, perceived by authorities in some cases as encouraging drug use.

Concerns about MDMA causing brain damage were raised when researcher George Ricaurte and colleagues gave monkeys a four-day course of MDMA. Two weeks later, there was evidence of some changes in serotonin receptors. Seven years later, the researchers found that the changes had not been reversed. It can be argued that this study was not done on Ecstasy-popping clubbers but on primates, and at very high doses. Moreover, the monkeys were in captivity, not in a natural environment, which also could have contributed to these findings. Nevertheless, these findings have serious implications that should not be ignored. More research needs to be done in this area. A recent study by Dr. Liesbeth Reneman and colleagues in the Netherlands found that there were long-term memory deficits in former MDMA users and that higher lifetime doses were related to greater deficits.

HUMAN STUDIES

Worries over long-term brain damage have been further fueled by research published in the *Lancet* in 1998. Brain scans of heavy Ecstasy users have shown damage to serotonin neurons caused, researchers believe, by MDMA. These were users of exceptionally high doses (average of 386 mg)—more than 200 times in fewer than five years. It is not possible to conclude that all the damage to serotonin neurons was caused by MDMA or that infrequent use results in the same kind of damage. In addition, not all studies have shown damage, and it certainly appears that damage is very dose-dependent.

In fact, similar changes have been seen in the brains of experimental animals given other serotonin-enhancing drugs, such as Prozac and Zoloft, in doses up to 100 times the normal human dose (by proportional body weight). The coauthor of the study, James O'Callahan, at the Center for Disease Control, as well as the manufacturer of Prozac, however, holds that these changes are unrelated to any physiological results and may not signify true damage. Thus, we can say only that either MDMA as well as the SSRIs in very high doses over time are causing "brain damage" or that MDMA's brain changes are not in the "dangerous" category.

In summary, evidence to date suggests that MDMA produces changes in serotonin-releasing neurons and may lead to serotonin deficiency. For a thorough discussion of the research, see "The Politics of MDMA Research" by UCLA's Dr. Charles Grob, reproduced on www.erowid.com.

In any case, most people report that MDMA not only "loses its magic" with repeated experiences but that there is an increase in negative side effects, such as depression and hangovers. So far, too, there has been little research into other reported concerns, including risks of cardiac arrhythmias, hypertension, strokes, and adverse drug interactions from MDMA use.

TO TAKE OR NOT TO TAKE?

The final verdict? Magic mushrooms, LSD, and Ecstasy are illegal. There is no quality control, so you may be taking something far more toxic than you expect. At best, it's a shortcut to achieving a temporary experience of enhanced perception and connection. Under the right circumstances, as with Jerome, it can be life-changing. The same can be said for the other entheogens as well. Frequent use has diminishing rewards, and possibly some risk of brain changes, the implications of which are still unclear.

You can see how this area is fraught with uncertainty and possible adverse effects. We can get you higher without the risks, and with completely natural nutrients and herbal connectors.

Natural Connectors: Be at One

You know those times when you feel completely in tune with others, and the world seems to be a wonderful place? No, it isn't the world that changes: it's the way you see it. And your perception is affected by both your brain's chemistry and your frame of mind. Entheogens such as Ecstasy (MDMA) can temporarily get you "high," but at a price. Natural connectors, on the other hand, combined with lifestyle changes that help develop the right frame of mind, can help you to feel connected much of the time, with no downside in sight.

In the following sections, we'll be investigating a handful of natural connectors that are widely available from supplement providers. Many of these substances were discussed earlier in the chapter on stress and relaxants, but you'll see that they also work as connectors:

- Tryptophan and 5-hydroxytryptophan (5-HTP).
- S-adenosyl-methionine (SAMe) and trimethylglycine (TMG).
- Vitamins B_3, B_6, B_{12}, and folic acid.
- Kava.
- Sceletium.

The chemistry of connection is all about having a healthy balance of neurotransmitters, specifically dopamine, serotonin, and DMT. The best way to achieve optimal levels is to supplement with a cocktail of supporting nutrients. Here's what happened to Jeremy, a psychologist who decided to try natural connectors:

> My life had become a roller coaster of highs and lows, with many more lows than highs. I decided to clean up my act for a month, and started taking 5-HTP, SAMe, and B vitamins, plus kava in the evenings. Within a week, I stopped feeling like a "victim" and started to feel in charge and in tune. My mood and outlook on life noticeably improved.

The amino acid tryptophan, found in protein foods such as milk and turkey, is the building block of both serotonin and DMT. In addition, the brain's chemistry is carefully and intelligently kept in order by catalysts, SAMe and B vitamins, that have the ability to change tryptophan into a number of natural connectors. They add or remove what are known as "methyl" groups. It has long been known that a deficiency in B vitamins can induce schizophrenia—the profound "dis-connection" of a person. These combinations of nutrients therefore help to fine-tune brain chemistry and allow for a more a natural and consistent state of connection.

TRYPTOPHAN AND 5-HTP (5-HYDROXYTRYPTOPHAN): CRUCIAL CONNECTORS

An adequate supply of tryptophan, combined with B vitamins, is critical to the chemistry of connection. We have seen how tryptophan deficiency leads to depression, impulsivity, and aggressiveness, while tryptophan supplementation is an effective antidepressant. In addition, a recent study showed that healthy volunteers given 1 g of tryptophan three times daily for twelve days showed an increase in their self-confidence and sociability and a decrease in quarrelsomeness. Meanwhile, the placebo group showed no such effect until the pills were switched. Only after the former placebo group was given tryptophan did it show the same positive changes.

Tryptophan is currently available only by prescription from special compounding pharmacies. (See Resources.) Because it competes with other amino acids for absorption into the brain, it is best taken with fruit or another carbohydrate snack. Avoid eating proteins an hour before or after taking it. See page 124 for dosage recommendations.

5-HTP: OVER-THE-COUNTER TRYPTOPHAN

5-HTP (5-hydroxytryptophan) is a more readily available form of tryptophan and may even be more biologically active. While not a direct precursor for DMT, it is the most effective precursor for serotonin. By providing the brain with the raw material to make serotonin, it spares tryptophan for production of other important tryptamines, such as DMT.

5-HTP can have profound mood-lifting effects, as Alex can attest:

I had recently ended a long-term relationship and was feeling lonely and a bit down, missing that company and connection. There were some good days when I felt fine, looking forward and getting on with life, but they were few and far between. Then I started taking 200 mg of 5-HTP a day. Within a couple of days, I felt much more "up," in the moment, and basically happier. I had more of an enjoyable, warm sense of detachment, that everything was all right, rather than a kind of gloomy seriousness. These days I don't take it all the time, but when I feel like I'm losing my balance, I include it in my daily supplement regime.

Here we have a temporary situation that might have lasted a lot longer if not for Alex's use of a natural connector and mood elevator. Why suffer needlessly when help is right there in a bottle? And remember, we are not talking about alcohol or other temporary escapes, but a truly restorative compound that produces lasting, positive effects.

Like tryptophan, 5-HTP has proven to be at least as effective as the best antidepressant drugs, but without the same high risk of side effects. 5-HTP occurs naturally in the African plant *Griffonia simplifica* and is available as a nutritional supplement.

Because 5-HTP doesn't compete for absorption with other amino acids, it is well absorbed, with or without food. The amount needed to promote a sense of connection is 100 mg a day, or less if taken in combination with other "connecting" nutrients, plus vitamin B_6. The dose range is one-tenth that of tryptophan.

A word of caution: more is not better. Serotonin overload can trigger serotonin syndrome—tremor, nausea, vomiting, elevated temperature, abnormal heartbeat, and, in extreme cases, coma, leading to death. It occurs within two hours, and symptoms subside within six to twenty-four hours. These side effects do not occur when taking the dose ranges we have suggested. We do not recommend simultaneously supplementing these nutrients with antidepressant drugs unless under medical guidance. The SSRIs effectively keep more serotonin in circulation by stopping its breakdown. Nor do we advise combining these nutrients with entheogens that temporarily raise serotonin levels. That being said, serotonin syndrome is still a rare occurrence, and has not been reported with either tryptophan or 5-HTP. See pages 124 and 126 for dosage guidelines.

SAMe (S-ADENOSYL-METHIONINE): THE MASTER TUNER

As far as the chemistry of connection is concerned, SAMe is the master tuner. It donates "methyl" groups to make naturally occurring tryptamines. By methylating tryptamine, for example, it produces DMT. The body makes SAMe from the amino acid methionine and the cofactor vitamins B_6, B_{12}, and folic acid.

SAMe also helps neurotransmitters deliver their messages to the receptor sites by sharpening their activity. By methylating phospholipids, from which nerve cell membranes are made, SAMe improves communication between nerve cells. SAMe also can help you get a good night's sleep and can promote dreaming. This is because the brain depends on SAMe to manufacture melatonin, a key neurotransmitter for sleep and dreaming, from serotonin.

A proven antidepressant, SAMe can also enhance a feeling of well-being and connection in "normal" folks. While a positive response is often felt within a week or sometimes within days, it may take as long as four weeks for overall mood elevation. In general, the longer SAMe is used, the more beneficial the results. For a "connection" experience for those with relatively normal brain chemistry, we have found that it can have an immediate effect.

SAMe should be taken on an empty stomach, preferably one hour before or after a meal, and at least 20 minutes before or after taking other supplements. Start with a dosage of 200 mg twice daily. If results aren't seen in a few days, you can gradually increase it, up to a maximum of 400 mg four times daily, if needed. Most often, 400 mg per day is sufficient. SAMe should also be taken with its cofactors, vitamins B_6 (100 mg), B_{12} (100 mcg), and folic acid (800 mcg), simply as part of your daily multivitamin regimen. It is safe to use during pregnancy and nursing.

A word of caution: although not reported in the literature, higher doses may lead to irritability and anxiety. If this continues, even on the lowest dose, stop taking SAMe. There are no reported negative interactions with other medications or nutritional supplements.

TMG (TRIMETHYLGLYCINE): CHEAP SAMe?

The body can make SAMe directly from TMG, which is more stable and much less expensive than SAMe, making it a reasonable substitute. While TMG has not been as extensively researched, the fact that it is a direct precursor of SAMe would predict that its effect would be similar. TMG also helps the body make more SAMe from dietary protein.

TMG is extracted from sugar beets and is also found in broccoli and spinach. Now, there's a reason to eat your greens! It has no reported side effects other than brief muscle-tension headaches if it is taken in large quantities without food. Optimal doses needed to raise SAMe levels in the body are 1,000–3,000 mg per day. In a combined formula, a 500-mg dose is sufficient.

SAMe (s-adenosyl-methionine) and TMG (trimethylglycine)

How they work: Naturally occurring methyl donors; essential in the manufacture of key brain chemicals such as DMT, serotonin, dopamine, and noradrenaline.

Positive effects: Enhance neurotransmitter activity; act as natural mood enhancers and stimulants; improve energy, mental clarity, and emotional balance, promoting natural connection.

Cautions: Higher doses may lead to irritability, anxiety, insomnia, and nausea. Taking SAMe with food decreases this possibility but may reduce the overall effect. SAMe's antidepressant activity may lead to the manic phase in individuals with bipolar disorder (manic depression).

Dosage: As a connector, 200–800 mg daily of SAMe between meals to promote absorption, *or* 500–3,000 mg daily of TMG. For depression dosage, see page 128.

Natural Highs

VITAMINS B$_3$, B$_6$, B$_{12}$, AND FOLIC ACID: A BRAIN'S BEST FRIENDS

B vitamins are the real workers in the enzymes that turn one brain chemical into another and keep you feeling happy and connected.

For some enzymes, you need vitamin B$_3$; for others, B$_6$, B$_{12}$, or folic acid. Not surprisingly, deficiency of any one of these vitamins leads to disconnection and is associated with depression, hallucinations, and schizophrenia. Schizophrenia is a mental illness marked by a sense of disconnection from the self, others, and reality. Supplementing with these B vitamins has the reverse effect, dramatically improving mental and emotional well-being.

As long ago as 1957, in the first double-blind study of its kind, Canadian psychiatrists Humphrey Osmond and Abram Hoffer proved that supplementing niacin normalized behavior in those diagnosed with schizophrenia. Dr. Hoffer, who is now in his eighties and is still actively practicing in Victoria, British Columbia, has treated more than 5,000 schizophrenic patients. He claims an 80 percent success rate using vitamin B$_3$ and other connector nutrients. (His definition of cure: free of symptoms and able to socialize and pay income tax!)

Hoffer and Osmond were also among the first scientists to investigate the chemistry of mescaline, the entheogen found in the peyote cactus. This research formed the basis for their theories on the use of nutrients to treat the mentally ill who suffer from frightening hallucinations. Their theories have proven correct, and, to this day, Hoffer believes an optimal intake of nutrients is essential to be mentally balanced as well as naturally high. Dr. Osmond also introduced author Aldous Huxley to mescaline, providing the inspiration for Huxley's famous book *The Doors of Perception* (from which Jim Morrison named his band, The Doors).

Meanwhile, Dr. Carl Pfeiffer at the Brain-Bio Center in Princeton had also been investigating the chemistry of the brain in relation to mental health and illness. He discovered that a deficiency in vitamin B$_6$ (pyridoxine) and zinc (pyridoxine is "activated" in the body by a zinc-dependent enzyme) also created schizophrenia. Supplementing vitamin B$_6$ and zinc corrected this abnormal chemistry and improved the mental health and experience of connection in people with schizophrenia.

Research at King's College Hospital and the Institute of Psychiatry in

London found that *one-third of all patients with either severe depression or schizophrenia were deficient in folic acid.* Supplementing folic acid for six months made a big difference in their symptoms and ability to relate. Folic acid, together with vitamin B$_{12}$, is needed to turn tryptophan into serotonin and tyrosine into dopamine. It appears, then, that without these vitamins, the higher brain centers simply can't work properly.

Of course, the effect of these nutrients in isolation is not nearly as powerful as they are in combination, and, consequently, it is best to supplement them daily to enhance connection.

Take B vitamins and minerals in the dosages noted below.

Niacin comes in two forms—niacin and niacinamide. At doses above 25–50 mg, niacin causes a flush. This effect is beneficial in many ways, but it's not to everyone's liking. Depending on your own response, supplement no more than 25–50 mg of niacin, and take the rest as niacinamide.

B Vitamins

How they work: Cofactors for making neurotransmitters; vital for enzymes that control the chemistry of connection; act as methyl group donors and acceptors.

Positive effects: Improve energy, memory, mood, and concentration; enhance connection; help to prevent the unpleasant hallucinations experienced in some types of schizophrenia.

Cautions: None when taken in sensible doses. Excess B$_3$ and B$_6$ can have adverse effects (above 1,000 mg a day). B$_3$ as niacin acts as a vasodilator, improving circulation and causing flushing at doses above 25–50 mg.

Daily Dosage: 25–50 mg of vitamin B$_3$ (niacin); 100 mg of niacinamide; 25–50 mg of vitamin B$_6$ (pyridoxine); 50–100 mcg of vitamin B$_{12}$ (cyanocobalamin); and 400–800 mcg of folic acid. Plus the following B vitamins for balance: 50 mg of vitamin B$_1$ (thiamine); 25 mg of vitamin B$_2$ (riboflavin); 50 mg of choline; and 50 mg of inositol.

The minerals below are necessary cofactors that help with the assimilation of the B vitamins.

Minerals	Daily Dose
Zinc	15–25 mg
Manganese	5–10 mg
Magnesium	400 mg

KAVA AS A CONNECTOR

While we have extolled the virtues of kava as a stress buster and natural relaxant (see Chapter 4), it certainly qualifies as a natural connector. Kava produces an experience of peace, relaxation, ease, well-being, and even euphoria. It opens you to an experience of heightened awareness and empathy, of enhanced "being," and of freedom from the usual mode of "doing." When you take kava, at least in the manner and doses used regularly in the South Pacific, your consciousness is unmistakably altered. It's difficult to improve on the description of anthropologist E. M. Lemert, who observed: "The head is affected pleasantly; you feel friendly, not beer sentimental; you cannot hate with kava in you. Kava quiets the mind; the world gains no new colour or rose tint; it fits in its place and in one easily understandable whole."

Referring to its subtlety, Islanders say, "Kava doesn't come to you. You go to kava." Terrence's description of his experience at a kava ceremony in Hawaii says it all:

Over the next several minutes, at least four things seem to happen fairly simultaneously. A wave of relaxation rolls through my body. The effects of kava are immediate, but they are not abrupt. The second thing is an emotional release, perhaps even more subtle than the phys-

ical. I don't notice the change as it happens, but I find I'm feeling at ease, comfortable in my skin, but again very awake.

Vision and hearing are slightly heightened. I've read of the Islanders' wanting silence and darkness because of increased sensitivity, but I've never found it uncomfortable. Both sights and sounds are just a little brighter, clearer, and warmer. Finally I'm aware of a feeling of easy connectedness and relationship with others in the room.

The potency of kava preparations varies, and the herb affects people differently. For some, kava's effects are too subtle; for others, too strong. Some people feel no effects the first couple of times they try kava. Others report feeling a little weird or sleepy at first, but with subsequent use, they experience a clearer, more pleasant state. It's as if the brain has to get used to a new sensation. This fogginess can also indicate underlying poor adrenal function, the result of excessive stress. A few tries will let you know which it is, and you can act accordingly. For the overly stressed, adrenal support is called for, as described in Chapter 4.

As we've noted, Pacific Islanders speak of "listening to kava." It opens a window to subtle awareness and a connection to nature, as well as to others and to oneself. Kava's first effects are felt within 30 minutes, and its mild high lasts two to three hours.

Kava has properties that clearly qualify it as an entheogen—increasing feelings of sociability, friendliness, and empathy toward others. One of the kavalactones, methysticin, actually bears some chemical similarity to MDMA, but kava would hardly be described as a hallucinogen. At most, some report that high doses of potent kava can cause mild visual and auditory distortions, such as objects taking on a subtle glow or a softness of focus.

You have to take relatively large amounts of the whole root to feel its mind-altering effects. One serving of the traditional island beverage, about half a cup, contains about 1,000 mg of resin, which equals about 250–500 mg of kavalactones. Islanders might consume five or more such servings in a single evening, for a total of 1,000–2,500 mg or more of kavalactones! Compare this to a typical tablet or capsule that contains only about 60–75 mg. You would have to take four to seven capsules for a serving, and the usual five servings would be at least twenty capsules or tablets! Tinctures wouldn't be any better. The only equivalent would be a traditional extract of ground kava powder, available in bulk at some herbal outlets or ethnic markets, or online. It's a messy business, but we do give instructions for those of you brave enough to try it. We also do not recommend the high doses taken by native drinkers.

With all due respect to the native liquid extraction process, we have found that you can attain the same elevated mood using store-bought capsules of known quality and potency, at doses of 60–250 mg of kavalactones.

Kava Beverage Recipes

If you are interested in preparing kava beverages from powder, two simple methods are described below: the water method and the emulsion method. Some of the resins in the root are extracted using just water. Others, which are not water soluble, need to be emulsified. The emulsion method should release more kavalactones.

Kava was traditionally ground and drunk fresh. In Fiji, dried kava—a result of commercialization—is known as "dead" kava, since it loses potency with grinding. Freeze-drying the resinous, milklike, non-water-soluble emulsion will preserve its freshness. Do not store the liquid, since, like milk, it is an environment for bacterial growth.

Remember: the powder extraction process is messy, has its own distinctive strong smell, and takes a little practice to master.

WATER METHOD

1 cup kava powder
4 cups water

Wrap kava powder loosely in a piece of cloth. Holding the edges of the cloth loosely above the ball of kava, plunge the kava up and down in the water, stopping occasionally to squeeze out the kava ball. Continue plunging it up and down until the water is a "coffee-and-cream" color. (This should take 5–15 minutes.) Drink!

EMULSION METHOD

1 cup kava powder
4 cups water
6 tablespoons vegetable oil (olive or canola)
2 tablespoons liquid lecithin

Blend all ingredients together in a blender at top speed for 5 minutes, until the liquid is a "coffee-and-cream" color. Strain liquid through a fiber filter. Since straining can take time (and patience), you may want to use something fairly loose, like cheesecloth. Eventually, all the liquid will drain out, leaving the solid ingredients in a ball in your strainer or cloth, and a bowl of suspicious-smelling liquid. Once this happens, you can throw away the solid mass. Enjoy!

KAVA COLADA

1 tray pineapple juice ice cubes
1 6-oz. to 8-oz. can coconut milk
1 fl oz kava extract
1 teaspoon honey
1 teaspoon vanilla

Blend all ingredients together in a blender at high speed until smooth. One or two of these smoothies will take your mind off your worries; stimulate thoughtful, authentic communication; and leave you feeling benevolent toward the world.

Yield: 6 servings
(Adapted from Chris Kilham's book *Psyche Delicacies*.)

Start low and work your way up. Kava is most potent when consumed on an empty stomach.

The danger of too much? You fall asleep and miss the whole experience. However, you will likely sleep deeply and well, and awake refreshed, with no hangover.

Those who do experience a hangover from kava should pay attention to their liver function, since it may indicate the liver's inability to fully break down the kavalactones. If this happens, take 200 mg of milk thistle (70 percent standardized) two to three times daily for a month or more to help support liver function. And have your liver status checked out by a health-care practitioner.

Kava definitely affects consciousness and thinking. In studies, memory actually seems to be enhanced. Perception is a bit heightened, and so is sensitivity to stimuli such as noises or bright lights. You're not likely to experience a loss of mental sharpness with kava, as you do with alcohol. (In some studies, kava actually enhanced mental sharpness.) But don't be fooled. Kava can deeply relax muscles, almost to the point of numbness. You can still function, but your coordination is impaired.

Definitely do not drive, operate heavy machinery, or care for young children under the too-relaxing influence of kava. Other than this, there appears to be no downside to using kava as a connector.

Kava

How it works: Appears to enhance GABA activity, the relaxing neurotransmitter that also modulates dopamine, adrenaline, and noradrenaline. (There is still much that is unknown about kava's effects on the brain.)

Positive effects: Heightened sensory perception, relaxation, well-being, connection, and empathy; effective antianxiety agent; promotes good sleep; muscle relaxant.

Cautions: Do not drive or operate heavy machinery after use; do not mix with alcohol, as the two substances seem to potentiate each other; do not take while using benzodiazepine tranquilizers. As with all herbs, do not take during pregnancy or while nursing.

Dosage: As a relaxant, 60–150 mg daily; as a connector, 60–250 mg daily.

SCELETIUM: SOUTH AFRICAN GEM

According to Dr. Nigel Gericke of African Natural Health in South Africa:

Sceletium is one of the most ancient of mind-altering substances, and it is likely to have had a profound influence on the evolution of human consciousness. People interested in consciousness will find that sceletium is a key, but it needs to be used widely. It is not a quick fix, and after ten years of use, I'm still learning about it.

Dr. Gericke is currently spearheading research into sceletium in cooperation with psychiatrists, including his wife, Dr. Olga Gericke, and psychologists in South Africa.

An unfamiliar herb to most of us, this native South African creeper, also called *kougoed,* has been used by hunter-gatherer tribes since prehistoric times. Sceletium is new to the American market and is only just starting to be manufactured here, so it may not be easy to find. It lessens anxiety, stress, and tension; raises spirits; and enhances the sense of connection. If you take a very large dose, you may even feel euphoric, then taken over by a sense of drowsiness. It does not cause hallucinations. Moreover, nearly 400 years of documented use have not revealed many serious adverse effects.

Traditionally, sceletium is chewed, brewed as a tea, or used as snuff. If enough is chewed, it has a mild anesthetic effect in the mouth, much like kava, and is used by the San people of South Africa for tooth extractions or is given in minute doses to children with colic. A tea made from sceletium is used to help the recovering alcoholic avoid withdrawal symptoms.

People have reported that sceletium-induced relaxation has helped them to focus on inner thoughts and feelings or to have a heightened experience of the beauty of nature. Some have reported increased skin sensitivity as well as sexual arousal, while others have said that it leaves them feeling free of fear and stress. In his 1934 book *Phantastica,* Dr. Louis Lewin reports that mesembrine—one of the active chemicals in the plant—induces a meditative state of mind.

While no clinical trials have been published yet, a number of doctors and psychiatrists have reported a wide range of positive uses for sceletium—

from treating anxiety and depression to alleviating alcohol, cocaine, and nicotine addiction. Moreover, by promoting a sense of empathy and connection, it has also been reported to help couples in therapy.

How does it work? The active constituents of the plant are alkaloids, including mesembrine, mesembrone, mesembrenol, and tortuosamine. According to laboratory studies sponsored by the National Institute of Mental Health near Washington, D.C., its major alkaloid, mesembrine, acts as a serotonin reuptake inhibitor. Like Prozac, it helps to keep more serotonin in circulation. It also appears to have a harmonizing and balancing effect on the other feel-good neurotransmitters, dopamine and norepinephrine, as well as on adrenaline.

Sceletium

How it works: Appears to enhance activity of serotonin, the mood-enhancing neurotransmitter; helps to balance dopamine, adrenaline, and noradrenaline. (There is still much that is unknown about its effects on the brain.)

Positive effects: Relieves depression, tension, and anxiety; promotes a sense of connection; associated with insights, heightened sensory perception, and improved meditation; also reduces addictive craving.

Caution: In very large doses, it can have euphoric effects, followed by sedation. Sceletium has not been researched sufficiently to recommend its use during pregnancy or nursing. No reported toxicity. However, we do not recommend taking it with antidepressants or with large amounts of tryptophan or 5-HTP, to avoid the possibility of serotonin syndrome—headache, an increase in body temperature, and heavy sweating (although this has never been reported). Stop taking it and seek medical advice if this occurs.

Dosage: As a mood enhancer, 50–100 mg daily; as a connector, 100–200 mg daily.

An effective dose is 50 mg a day, although some doctors prescribe 100–200 mg a day for those with chronic depression or anxiety.

Twenty-eight-year-old Alex is a new advocate of sceletium. Here's what he has to say:

> *I used to drink on Friday nights to unwind after my stressful week. Now I prefer sceletium. I combine 100 mg of sceletium with 75 mg of kava and 500 mg of TMG. This not only chills me out but it makes me feel very connected and "present" and able to really enjoy my friends' company. It's a bit like the buzz you get sitting on the beach watching the waves rolling in. What's more, there's no hangover.*

ACTION PLAN FOR GETTING CONNECTED

The first step to feeling connected naturally is to tune up all your neurotransmitters. In other words, follow all the advice so far. This includes reducing your stress level, eating well, balancing your blood sugar, and reducing your intake of stimulants to an absolute minimum. A good all-around multivitamin/mineral is key. Also, Part Three will give you advice on exercises and lifestyle changes that will promote your sense of connection.

The nutrients listed in the following chart are worthy additions to a supplement program designed to enhance connection. This combination, taken every day, is likely to improve meditation, dreaming, insights, and understanding, as well as your mood and ability to relate. While the daily dose may seem complex, the good news is that there are ready-made formulas available that contain various combinations of these substances. (See the Resources section at the back of the book.) The ideal doses of the "connector nutrients" are less when combined than when a substance is taken in isolation.

You may want to begin with 60–75 mg of kava, especially if you tend to have some level of anxiety or irritability, and double the dose if necessary.

So, to sum up, you should take the following to get connected:

A good all-around multivitamin and mineral formula supplying optimal amounts of the B vitamins and the minerals zinc, manganese, and magnesium.

A "connector nutrient" formula providing 5-HTP, SAMe, or TMG; kava; and additional B vitamins to achieve the levels shown above. SAMe is best supplemented separately.

For a full natural program promoting feelings of connection, see Top Tips in Part Four.

Daily Doses for Getting Connected
(Divide into two to three doses daily.)

L-tryptophan	500–3,000 mg
5-HTP*	50–300 mg
SAMe+	40–800 mg
or	
TMG	500–3,000 mg
Kava (standardized extract)**	60–250 mg
Sceletium	100–200 mg
Vitamin B_3 (niacin)	25–50 mg
Niacinamide	100 mg
Vitamin B_6 (pyridoxine)	25–50 mg
Vitamin B_{12} (cyanocobalamin)	50–100 mcg
Folic acid	400–800 mcg

*Do not supplement 5-HTP with antidepressant medication. One supplies the precursor to make serotonin, while the other prevents the breakdown of serotonin. Taking both could lead to serotonin overload. Don't exceed this amount if combining with sceletium.

+SAMe can be substituted by its precursor, TMG, which is more stable and less expensive.

**The kava dosage given here relates to the actual amount of kavalactones in the product, be it powder, capsules, or tincture.

9

"Addicted? I Can Quit
Whenever I Want"

- Do you sneak candy bars and then hide the wrappers so others won't find out?
- Do you crave your first morning cup of coffee, or *really* look forward to your coffee break?
- Do you find you can't wait to get home for that after-work drink, and can't relax without it?
- Are you secretive about the amount you smoke?

You are not alone. Here is a story that may seem familiar, if not to you, then to someone you know:

> Margo, a thirty-five-year-old stewardess, came into the office for a "tune-up." She noticed that she was more tired and less able to adapt to time-zone changes than in the past. When asked to describe her diet, she was quick to warn, "Don't make me give up my drink with dinner!"

This big attachment to a habit is often a clue that some degree of dependency is involved. (If alcohol had held no charge for her, she wouldn't

189

have even thought of mentioning it. We're not talking about the one drink a day, but about the attitude.) And she could just as easily have said "coffee" or "dessert." The trick now was for her to change her relationship to drinking.

It was important to avoid the "A" word, for "alcohol," at this point. That is, if Margo did decide to stop, it would be by choice, and with no guilt or suffering, either. With the right nutrients, cravings can be stopped quickly and often painlessly.

Margo began a supplement program that included 500–1,000 mg of the amino acid L-glutamine at the times when she would usually consider a drink. Sure enough, she noticed that she no longer was craving a glass of wine. Before long, she could barely even identify with the Margo that had. This convenient "forgetting" is an interesting phenomenon that psychotherapists see over and over again.

"Who me? I don't remember doing that!"

When people correct an emotional issue, or even a physical symptom, they often develop a sort of amnesia about it. It is as if the "normal" person one becomes no longer has the space to carry around the formerly unbalanced self. The old behaviors and relationships are replaced with healthier ones. Like Margo, this healthier person no longer lives in the damage of the past. Margo's experience is a tribute to the ability of the human being to grow beyond adversity and to flower. One leaves behind the old self, like a butterfly leaving its cocoon and its prior existence as a caterpillar. It is history.

The Hidden Addiction

When someone like Margo has a problem with a substance, it's usually not that they are weak-willed. They simply have an underlying chemical imbalance. And this imbalance can be depleting their energy and peace of mind, and they don't even know it!

Now you may protest, "but I just *like* my morning coffee" . . . (or "my after-work beer with my friends" . . . or "my glass of wine with dinner" . . .). I could give it up any time." And often these habits appear to be just tension relievers, pick-me-ups, or one of the normal pleasures of life. But are they? Generally not, and we'll will tell you why. You can then apply this to your own life, and see what fits.

Research shows that we can successfully treat addiction with the use of specific amino acids. These include precursors to the neurotransmitters serotonin, dopamine, and glutamine, as well as GABA (a neurotransmitter *and* amino acid).

When neurotransmitter precursors were given to alcoholic subjects, the individuals experienced:

- Fewer cravings for alcohol.
- Reduced incidence of stress.
- Increased likelihood of recovery.
- Reduction in relapse rates.

How many programs can boast that record? And willpower has nothing to do with it! To prove the point, similar research has been done with rats, where they were made "alcoholic," then treated with amino acids. When tested further, they had lost their cravings and addiction!

Addicted to Carbs

It's not only alcohol that is addictive. Food addiction, to carbohydrates in particular, is a major issue for many people, especially women, as we see here:

On the surface, Kim's situation was not unusual. A successful thirty-eight-year-old professional, she was a single working mother of two energetic teenagers and found herself with an ever-growing list of unfinished tasks. Exhausted and near burnout, she felt stretched emotionally, financially, and professionally. She would "collapse into bed in a heap" at night and fall asleep easily. However, she would often awaken at 3 or 4 A.M., her heart pounding, her mind racing, and unable to fall back to sleep until just before the alarm rang at 6:30. It didn't matter what time she went to bed, either.

Kim's diet was fast food, doughnuts, and coffee, consumed on the run. She suffered from frequent headaches, heart palpitations, and, at times, shakiness. Her symptoms pointed to hypoglycemia, which can appear in many forms: depression, irritability, anxiety, panic attacks, fatigue, "brain fog," headaches (including migraines), insomnia, muscular weakness, and tremors. All of these symptoms may be relieved by food. Cravings can be for sweets, coffee, alcohol, or drugs; in fact, many addictions are related to hypoglycemia.

When Kim ate high glycemic foods, such as doughnuts and candy, or drank coffee, her blood-sugar levels rose rapidly. This led to a large, fast release of insulin, which then removed the sugar from circulation, storing it as fat and glycogen. This caused her blood-sugar levels to drop over the next one to two hours, making Kim feel weak, lightheaded, and even cranky. When this cycle repeated itself enough, the overtaxed adrenal glands became exhausted—and so did she.

THE SOLUTION

To support Kim's adrenals and balance her blood sugar, she was given the following recommendations:

Kim implemented *dietary changes,* including the elimination of refined carbohydrates, such as sugar and white flour, as well as cutting out coffee and alcohol. She made an effort to eat small, frequent meals containing protein and complex carbohydrates, which have a low glycemic index (see pages 32–35 in Chapter 3). This index measures how quickly a specific food is turned into glucose, or blood sugar, which in turn stimulates the pancreas to release insulin.

The result? Vegetables and whole grains allowed for more stable blood-sugar levels, which increased Kim's energy and her ability to handle stress. The complex carbohydrates also helped raise her serotonin levels, which both calmed her down and lifted her mood. Serotonin is sensitive to shifts in female hormones, explaining the sugar cravings that often accompany PMS.

SUPPLEMENTS

Kim was given a daily nutritional supplement regimen. This included a high-potency multivitamin and mineral formula for basic support, containing at least 75 mg of each of the B vitamins and 200 mg of chromium to help balance blood sugar; 400 mg of magnesium; 10 mg of manganese; 500–1,000 mg of potassium; and 15–30 mg of zinc. In addition, she was given 2 g of pantothenic acid (vitamin B_5) and 3,000 mg of vitamin C; and for cravings, 500–1,000 mg of glutamine, as needed. This works for most cravings, since it raises brain glucose. She also needed 100 mg of 5-HTP twice a day to raise her serotonin levels.

EXERCISE

Kim began to exercise regularly, which allowed her to burn fat, maintain blood-sugar levels, relieve anxiety, and elevate her mood. Regular exercise can actually reduce the amount of adrenal hormones the body releases in response to stress. In addition, it raises the level of the mood-elevating hormones, or endorphins, in the brain.

RESULTS

Kim's new habits had a marked effect on stabilizing her mood. Her physical symptoms cleared, too. There were no more early morning awakenings, no more headaches, and no more fatigue. The stresses of life as a busy mother and office worker continued, but she no longer fell victim to her inner chemistry. She now had an internal buffer against stress—functioning adrenal glands and a smoother supply of blood sugar to her body, particularly to her brain.

The predisposition to hypoglycemia runs in families, so if you are prone, you need to be more attentive to stress, diet, and nutritional supplements. Relaxation techniques are useful, too, and once balance is restored, psychotherapy can be helpful in revealing and dealing with the underlying dynamics.

Are You a Stimulant Addict?

Take another look at the questions at the beginning of this chapter and the Energy Check questionnaire on page 14. If this sounds like you, you'll need to assess your current relationship to stimulants. All you need to do is keep a daily diary, just for three days. Mark down how much and when you consume coffee, tea, chocolate, sugar (or something sweet), cigarettes, or alcohol. And note how intensely you crave them.

Coffee-craving patients are often hypoglycemic, and you may suffer from poor adrenal or thyroid function. The solution is a good diagnostic evaluation, with treatment as necessary—improved diet, exercise, and specific supplements. When hypoglycemic people reduce their dependence on caffeine, they find that their overall energy levels rise.

STIMULANT ADDICTION AND BREAKING FREE

Now let's look at stimulants in action—how they can addict you and how to break free.

Jonathan, a thirty-two-year-old sales agent, had been a cocaine addict for several years. He explained how, "after years of depression and no motivation, using the drug actually made me feel normal for the first time in my life!" He also drank too much and had some other extreme behaviors. He had destroyed his marriage through compulsive casual sex with other women and was heavily in debt from excessive gambling. Jonathan raised his brain's feel-good chemicals with both cocaine and the adrenaline rush of thrill-seeking, risky behaviors. The problem? He was requiring increasing amounts of everything just to stay even, and his life was falling apart around him. The solution? Jonathan explains:

> Fortunately, with the support of Gamblers Anonymous and Co-caine Anonymous, I was able to pull myself out of this mess, and recover some self-esteem. I started taking some vitamins that helped with my energy and cravings. I finally found the job I'm in—it's been three years now—and I have been clean the whole time. No drugs,

alcohol, gambling, or chasing after women. I realized that those "bored" feelings were depression, and the coke and alcohol made me feel normal, at least briefly. I've been helped enormously by vitamins, the 12-step programs, eating right, and exercising regularly.

I don't even drink coffee or use sugar—I found that they were as addictive as drugs, and would give me the same pattern of highs and lows. My ADD (attention deficit disorder) is under control, too. I can concentrate, remember things, and keep my desk and my life organized for the first time. It's been a hard road, but I can honestly say that I have never felt better! Let me tell you, drugs just aren't worth it. I've been there and back, and I know.

What was Jonathan's problem? Moral weakness? Poor upbringing? Bad luck? Knowing the source of the problem helps us to find the solution. As it turned out, Jonathan was suffering from what researcher Dr. Kenneth Blum has termed *the reward deficiency syndrome (RDS)*. People with RDS are born with a tendency toward low moods and have difficulty feeling "normal." While extreme, Jonathan's out-of-control addiction to cocaine, gambling, alcohol, fast living, and high-risk behavior helps us to understand the full range of the problem. He had a biological tendency toward RDS (low levels of certain key neurotransmitters), and once he started using drugs, he couldn't stop. Even in "normal" people, repeated use of certain substances can lead to addiction, as can stress itself.

TREATMENT ISSUES

Jonathan's only escape was to gradually stop using the addictive substances. By taking natural supplements, he was able to restore chemical balance and end his cravings. With adequate neurotransmitter precursors, such as DLPA, L-glutamine, and tyrosine, 500 mg of each three times daily, his mood became normal, without the depression and anxiety that he had always plagued him.

You may wonder how he could overcome a biological and, most likely, genetic problem, and with such low-tech medicine. Here's the answer: We are not simply victims of our genetic makeup. Genetics give only the *predis-*

position to a condition. Its actual manifestation, or *expression,* can be influenced and changed. Jonathan was thus able to take measures, as can you, to control how these genes were expressed; that is, how they actually affected him. By understanding our propensities, we can take the appropriate precautionary steps or do good remedial work if we have already been affected.

This model applies to the use of caffeine, sugar, chocolate, and tobacco, as well. Each has its own way of stimulating the reward cascade, but the end result is the same. Blood sugar and dopamine are raised, and the brain becomes addicted to them. This cycle is often quite subtle.

Treatment Options from Dr. Cass

I see a variety of patients who are already in various stages of recovery from alcohol, cocaine, pot, opiates, and so on. But, in all cases, the treatment is similar. The good news is, you don't have to "power through" it. There are ways to cut the cravings to a minimum, by taking the right supplements and, when possible, by using techniques such as NAET discussed in the next section. As in Margo's case, I may not even have to address the problem head-on. I learned this early in my career in nutritional psychiatry, and rather by accident.

Bruce, a thirty-five-year-old realtor with a high pressure, competitive job, came to see me for anxiety, depression, and low energy. His intake questionnaire revealed that he drank a six-pack of beer every two days or so. Ignoring that specific issue, we began several sessions of counseling, including stress-reduction techniques such as meditation.

I also prescribed a series of supplements to address his physiological imbalances, including a daily high-potency, high–B vitamin multivitamin and mineral formula, 200 mcg of chromium daily for blood-sugar balance, 500–1,000 mg of tyrosine twice daily for energy, and 500 mg of glutamine three times a day for low mood and substance cravings. When I asked two months later about his beer drinking, he first gave me a blank look, then lit up and exclaimed, "Funny you should ask. I just noticed a six-pack that had been sitting in the refrigerator for weeks, untouched, and wondered why I had it there."

With Bruce, as with Margo, not only do the habits disappear, but so does the memory of their having been there.

Unblocking Energy Flow with NAET

Another technique that is very helpful in changing people's relationships to their addictive substances is called Nambudripad's Allergy Elimination Technique (NAET), named for the Southern California doctor who developed it. NAET employs a diagnostic method called "applied kinesiology." The practitioner uses an indicator muscle, like the shoulder (deltoid) muscle, and pushes down on the person's arm while the subject is holding a substance extract (usually in a tiny glass vial) in the other hand to determine if it causes his or her energy to strengthen or weaken. The craved substances are actually poorly tolerated by the body and therefore weaken it, but they are needed to stave off withdrawal. You can try this test yourself with a friend. For example, say, "My name is X" (give your real name). Your muscle should remain strong and able to resist the downward push. Then say, "My name is George" (unless it really is!) and have your friend test your muscle strength again. You should be significantly weaker, and your arm will go down. You can also test for allergies to various foods this way.

Acupressure is a good compliment to NAET. Once the substance that is weakening the subject has been identified, strategically placed acupuncture needles can release energy blocks and reprogram the brain to stop identifying the substance as an allergen. The end result is that the inner imbalances related to the substance are corrected, and the craving is gone or markedly reduced, often permanently. For allergenic foods, a patient can often resume eating them a day or so after treatment without further problems.

With the "bad stuff," such as alcohol or drugs, being able to resume their use is not the goal. Those substances will always be toxic to the body. We can remove only the craving with this technique, not the intrinsic toxicity of the product. While all this may sound strange or similar to a "placebo effect," the positive results are compelling. Remember, Westerners were quite skeptical of acupuncture (and its offshoot, acupressure) when they first heard of it, but now it has become a mainstream practice. NAET and related methods such as BioSet, developed by Dr. Ellen Cutler, are practiced successfully by many health-care practitioners. To find a practitioner in your area, visit www.naet.org or www.drellencutler.com.

Overcoming Addiction

The trick to overcoming addiction is to restore and regulate normal neuro-transmitter balance, and even, maybe, *have* balance for the first time. In this section, we will look at the most common addictive substances—cigarettes, sugar, caffeine, alcohol—and how to break free.

TIPS FOR HANDLING CRAVINGS

Take a 500-mg capsule of L-glutamine, open it, and pour the powdered contents under your tongue. It is absorbed quickly and should give you a pick-me-up similar to that of your longed-for stimulant, including alcohol. You can also take a 500-mg capsule of L-glutamine several times a day, be-tween meals, to prevent cravings. Adding 500 mg of DL-phenylalanine, two to three times daily, will also give you a desired energy boost.

Sugar Cravings
Although we are born with a liking for sweet things, sugar is an acquired taste. Research has shown that children who are fed sweet foods (cakes, pies, cook-ies, chocolate, candy, sweetened soft drinks, and so on) prefer higher levels of sweetness as adults. So as you gradually cut down the level of sweetness in *all* the food you eat, you will soon grow accustomed to the taste. Try to sweeten cereals and desserts with fruit, and if you're really desperate, have a sugar-free fruit-and-nut bar from your local health food store. Don't use sugar substitutes, since they don't allow you to change your habits. Do check la-bels for the many forms of sugar (fructose, corn syrup, and so on) and pur-chase those items with the lowest amounts or, better yet, with none at all.

Meanwhile, shift to a hypoglycemic diet to help maintain your blood sugar naturally (see Chapter 3). You will be amazed at how the desire for your sugar fix disappears. And take the supplements recommended on page 44.

Chocolate Cravings
Among other ingredients, chocolate contains phenethylamine (PEA), mag-nesium, fat, and sugar. One of these ingredients is probably causing your craving. If you can't figure out which it is, take the following supplements to cover all four: 500–1,000 mg of DL-phenylalanine two to three times

daily; 400–600 mg of magnesium daily; 1 tablespoon of flaxseed or hemp oil twice daily; and the supplements recommended for sugar cravings.

Coffee and Caffeine Cravings

It takes an average of four days to break the coffee habit. During this time, you may experience headaches and drowsiness. These are strong reminders of how bad coffee really is for you. Decaffeinated coffee contains less caffeine, but it is only mildly better than the caffeinated type. A delicious natural coffee alternative is grain-based Teeccino, available at many health food stores and by mail order. When brewed, it even tastes like the real thing. Visit www.teeccino.com for more information.

Tea Cravings

Try a lower caffeine tea, and green tea, then move on to caffeine-free herbal teas. Green tea isn't caffeine-free, but it has much less caffeine than regular tea and has other health benefits. See page 107 for more information on green tea.

Alcohol Cravings

It is all too easy to overindulge in alcohol because of its role in social interaction. Start by limiting the times you have alcohol. For instance, cut out your lunchtime drink. (You'll certainly work better in the afternoon.) Ideally, cut it out completely for at least two weeks. If you find this hard to do, take a close look at your drinking habits and, if necessary, seek professional help.

There is a great deal of self-deception that goes on in the name of "just social drinking." Some signs: your friends or spouse tells you that you drink too much; you have been arrested for driving while under the influence of alcohol; you look forward to dinner because it's preceded by a martini. Be especially concerned if alcoholism runs in your family. Above all remember: this is a brain imbalance, not a crime, but it can turn into one if you don't do something about quitting.

DETOXIFY YOUR BODY

One factor that helps to reduce cravings is boosting the body's ability to detoxify and eliminate stored chemicals, including nicotine. There are sev-

Lucy's Freedom from Alcohol Addiction

Lucy sent me the following e-mail, two months after I suggested that she try glutamine for her alcohol addiction:

I've had three wonderfully clean weeks since you gave me the name of the "magical" powder. I waited all this time because it didn't seem possible, but it was *immediate*. For me, it was a miracle!

I've lost 10 lbs. I lost my daily morning cough. My complexion is so much clearer. I have 4–6 more hours of daily LIFE.

Best of all, I feel like a different person, with a new personality. So I thank you very much . . . my life is changed. *I stand still and study my body to see why I don't crave a drink . . . is it in my brain?* Why don't AA and the CDC and all the doctors know about this magic over-the-counter item?

Lucy's weight loss was a "side benefit," since glutamine reduces carb cravings by raising brain blood sugar. Her clearer complexion was likely due to the glutamine, an effective healing agent for the lining of the gastrointestinal tract, often inflamed in alcoholics.

eral things you can do to speed up this process: perform sweat-producing exercises and activities, drink plenty of water, and supplement with vitamin C and niacin. Put these all together, and you've got a winning formula for rapid detoxification.

If you have access to a sauna or steam room, here's what you should do. (Most gyms have one or the other. This is a great excuse to enroll in a regular exercise program at your local gym.)

1. Take 1 g of vitamin C and 100 mg of niacin about 15 minutes before beginning activity.
2. Run or undertake any cardiovascular exercise that raises your pulse rate and stimulates circulation for about 30 minutes.
3. Once you begin to experience the niacin flush, enter the sauna or steam room. (The sauna should never be at a temperature above 80°F, or 27°C.)
4. Have a quart of water with you and drink it at regular intervals.

5. Remain in the sauna or steam room for 20 to 30 minutes. At any sign of faintness, leave the sauna.
6. Shower.

Do this every day for seven days. This routine is *not* recommended for those with a history of cardiovascular disease except under medical supervision.

HOW TO QUIT SMOKING

Nicotine is more addictive than heroin, which makes quitting smoking difficult. Even in small doses, nicotine produces a substantial effect. It can give you a lift, curb your appetite, and, at tense times, a puff can relax you.

All of these effects are due to nicotine's action on adrenal hormones, blood sugar, and brain chemicals. By following the "Natural High Diet" in Chapter 3, the craving for cigarettes will diminish as you stabilize your blood-sugar and hormone levels. So, before you even begin to try to quit cigarettes, we recommend following these diet and supplement guidelines for a month or so, until you no longer consume any other stimulants (such as tea, coffee, and chocolate) or sugar. Instead, you'll be eating small, frequent meals, with an emphasis on foods containing slow-releasing carbohydrates combined with foods rich in protein.

You are likely addicted to smoking at particular times, such as when you are tired, hungry, or upset; upon waking; with a drink after a meal; or after sex. Note what these cues are, and cut them out, one by one. You will be left with "just smoking."

Then reduce your nicotine load gradually by switching to brands that contains less nicotine, until the cigarettes you smoke contain no more than 2 mg of nicotine per cigarette. In addition to the supplements recommended in Chapter 3, take the following daily:

- 1,000 mg of vitamin C.
- 100 mcg of chromium.
- 50 mg of niacin. You may experience a flushing sensation 15 to 30 minutes after taking niacin. The flush will last about 15 minutes. It helps to take niacin with a meal.

- 600 mg of calcium and 400 mg of magnesium. Both are alkaline minerals that help to neutralize the excess acidity that adds to the craving.
- 2 tablespoons of lecithin granules.
- 200 mg of 5-hydroxytryptophan (5-HTP), either 100 mg twice daily or 200 mg one hour before bed, since serotonin levels rise at night and promote sleep. (Nicotine withdrawal tends to lower serotonin levels, leaving you depressed and irritable.)

HELPFUL HINTS

Meditation, deep breathing, and the other activities covered in Part Three are very useful for all addictions. In addition, after a session or two of flotation in an isolation tank, people often find that their cravings disappear. Regular aerobic exercise also helps, so this is a great time to sign up at your local gym, start jogging, or do the exercises in Chapter 11. And, finally, acupuncture is a great adjunct to any withdrawal and detoxification program.

To sum up, here are some practical steps for breaking addictions to stress and stimulants:

- Identify the stimulants that you are addicted to.
- Follow the "Natural High Diet" in Chapter 3.
- Avoid sugar and high-glycemic foods.
- Reduce your intake of stimulants by finding which substitutes you like the most until they are no longer a daily requirement.
- Notice your patterns of stressful behavior and replace them with a more positive response.
- Integrate the mind-body techniques in Part Three into your life.

Coming off Prescription Medications

If you take antianxiety drugs, you have a lot of company. More than 4 million Americans take prescription benzodiazepines such as Valium or Xanax every day, often for years. Two-thirds of benzodiazepine prescriptions are written by family practitioners and the remainder by psychiatrists. A good guide to this problem is Dr. Edward Drummond's book *Overcoming Anxiety Without Tranquilizers*.

Though less generally recognized, there are also withdrawal effects from antidepressants, especially the SSRIs (selective serotonin reuptake inhibitors)—Prozac, Zoloft, Paxil, and Celexa. First, however, we will examine withdrawal from benzodiazepines.

MINIMIZING BENZODIAZEPINE WITHDRAWAL SYMPTOMS WITH NATURAL REMEDIES

Coming off benzodiazepines has its own hazards and must be done under medical supervision. Abrupt withdrawal from high doses can lead to seizures or even death. Remember Marcy's case on page 58? She was hooked on Valium and finally took herself off it, cold turkey. Not a good idea. If you recall, she had many of the usual withdrawal symptoms: insomnia, anxiety, irritability, sweating, blurred vision, diarrhea, tremors, mental impairment, and headaches. Had she known better, she would have gone on a gradual program of withdrawal coupled with natural remedies such as kava and valerian, which can ease and shorten the transition phase.

The ideal withdrawal program has to be tailored to each individual's unique circumstances—the amount of the drug taken, the length of use, and the person's unique physiology. It takes months to get off these drugs completely, and professional support and guidance are essential.

As we've said, valerian (see page 70) is a great help in the process of withdrawal. A GABA enhancer, it will have similar actions to the drug but is much gentler and doesn't have the same addictive potential. The same is true for kava (see page 64). You gradually reduce the tranquilizer dose while increasing that of either (or both) valerian and kava. Experiment with each, and see which one works for you. Each has its own actions and "feel," so the choice depends on how well it's doing the job.

A word of caution: Since benzodiazepines, kava, and valerian all enhance GABA, the combination of the herbs with tranquilizer drugs can make the drugs' effects more potent. This point of caution is made in the German government's Commission E Report, a common reference manual on the use of herbal medicines. It recommends care when combining kava with any psychoactive substance, which would include benzodiazepines. For this reason, valerian and kava should be viewed in the same way as any medicine and taken in carefully scheduled doses as part of a medically supervised withdrawal program. In other words, you should not just add them in yourself. It is also helpful to add supplements that support the liver's ability to detoxify these drugs, such as milk thistle *(Silymarin silibum),* a liver-enhancing herb to speed up the breakdown of these drugs in your body. Since the herbs are not addictive and do not build tolerance, you don't have to be weaned off them later.

The dose range for valerian is 50–100 mg two to three times daily. For kava, we recommend 60–120 mg of kavalactones two to three times daily, modified according to where you are in the detox process. If combining the two, take into consideration the total effect of the two herbs and adjust these doses accordingly. You also need 200 mg of milk thistle (standardized to 70 percent silymarin complex) twice a day to help the detoxification process.

To sum up, here are some practical steps to take to break addiction to benzodiazepines and to minimize symptoms of withdrawal:

- Undertake a detoxification program only under the guidance of a physician.
- Deal with any psychological issues with the guidance of a psychotherapist.
- Start with milk thistle to support the liver, then gradually reduce the tranquilizer dose, under professional guidance, and replace with valerian and/or kava.
- When withdrawal symptoms are gone, reduce the dose of valerian and/or kava.
- Follow the dietary guidelines in Chapter 3 throughout the process.

SSRI WITHDRAWAL

Increasingly, information is coming to light about withdrawal problems with the SSRI antidepressants. Experts assert that, technically, SSRIs are not ad-

Addiction Is a Brain Disease

The director of the National Institute on Drug Abuse (NIDA), Dr. Alan Leshner, notes in the *Journal of the American Medical Association (JAMA)* (Oct. 13, 1999), "Advances in science have greatly increased, and in fact revolutionized, our fundamental understanding of the nature of drug abuse and addiction, and, most importantly, what to do about it.

"Although the onset of addiction begins with the voluntary act of taking drugs, the continued repetition of 'voluntary' drug taking begins to change into 'involuntary' drug taking, ultimately to the point where the behavior is driven by compulsive craving for the drug. This compulsion results from a combination of factors, including in large part dramatic changes in brain function produced by prolonged drug use. This is why addiction is considered a brain disease—one with imbedded behavioral and social context aspects. Once addicted, it is almost impossible for most people to stop the spiraling cycle of addiction on their own without treatment."

dictive. However, whatever we want to call it, there are definite issues of tolerance and withdrawal that must be addressed. In his book *Prozac Backlash,* Harvard psychiatrist Joseph Glenmullen begins by describing the ominous long-term side effects associated with these serotonin-boosting medications. These include neurological disorders, such as facial and whole-body tics (tardive dyskinesia) that can indicate brain damage; sexual dysfunction in up to 60 percent of users; debilitating withdrawal symptoms, including visual hallucinations, electric shocklike sensations in the brain, dizziness, nausea, and anxiety; and a decrease of antidepressant effectiveness in about 35 percent of long-term users. In addition, his research points to the direct link between these drugs and suicide and violence. For more information, visit www.glenmullen.com.

Unless patients are warned to come off these drugs very slowly by shaving minuscule amounts off their pill each day, as opposed to cutting them in half or taking a pill every other day, they can go into withdrawal, which can last for several months. Symptoms include bouts of overwhelming depression, insomnia, and fatigue and can include life-threatening physical effects, psychosis, or violent outbursts. Many psychiatrists cavalierly minimize these problems.

This chart summarizes what you have learned in Part Two. Check applicable feelings and the substances you use. This will show you the "natural solution" you need to restore your brain chemistry balance.

Supplement Directory

FEELING	COMMONLY USED SUBSTANCES	DEFICIENT NEUROTRANSMITTER	NATURAL SOLUTION
Stressed:			
Irritable	Sweets	**GABA Serotonin**	GABA
Worried	Chocolate	for emotional stability,	Taurine
Stressed, tense	Alcohol	self-confidence	Kava
Headaches	Tobacco		Valerian
Sleep problems	Marijuana		Hops
	Tranquilizers		Passionflower
Low Energy:			
Depressed	Caffeine	**Dopamine**	Tyrosine
Bored	Tobacco	**Noradrenaline**	DLPA
Tired	Chocolate	for energy, alertness,	*Adaptogens:*
Poor focus	Cocaine	mental focus,	Ginseng
Lack concentration	Speed	drive, motivation	Ashwaganda
Seek drama, thrills			Reishi mshrm
			Rhodiola
Depressed:			
Blue, sad	Sweets	**Serotonin**	5-HTP
Sleep problems	Chocolate	**Endorphins**	L-tryptophan

Depressed (continued)			
Fearful, hopeless	Alcohol	**Dopamine**	St. John's wort
Can't make decisions	Tobacco	**Noradrenaline**	SAMe
Evening cravings	Marijuana		TMG
Weight loss	Caffeine		
Overeating	Speed		
Low self-esteem	Antidepressants		

Brain Decline			
Declining memory/ mental abilities	Any of the above	**Acetylcholine**	Choline,
		Blood supply	Acetylcholine,
Absentminded		Oxygen	phosphatidylserine
Forget names, faces		Nutrients	DMAE
Mental fatigue			Ginkgo
Poor learning			Vinpocetine
Repeat self			EHA/DHA

Disconnected			
Bored	Alcohol	**Serotonin**	Kava
Life has no meaning	Marijuana	**Dopamine**	5-HTP
Isolated, lonely	Ecstasy	**Noradrenaline**	L-tryptophan
No spiritual connection	Psychedelics	**Endorphins**	SAMe
			Sceletium

Mood/Energy Swings			
Irritable, shaky between meals	Sweets, starch	**Serotonin**	L-glutamine
	Alcohol	Brain fuel	

Part Three

LIVING HIGH

NATURALLY

10

Living High Naturally

In the last part, we described how to shift our balance by using natural alternatives. We should not forget, however, that the real focus is in the
brain, where we actually manufacture our own neurotransmitters. That is,
while caffeine can stimulate us, it does so only by affecting the brain's production of dopamine. Similarly, we say that Valium or kava relax us, but the
real effect is caused in the brain by our very own GABA. We also produce
endorphins—morphinelike neuropeptides that relieve pain, enhance immunity, and make us feel euphoric.

Here, in Part Three, we will introduce you to other key aspects of
the Natural High equation that will help you to balance your own neurotransmitters and stay high naturally. We will examine techniques and lifestyle changes that will help you stay relaxed, alert, productive, and in high
spirits.

By understanding and incorporating the activities presented in the following chapters into your lifestyle, you will learn how to self-regulate your
mental and emotional states. The following is a good illustration of how one

young man combined supplements and self-regulation techniques to fine-tune his emotions, with great results:

When Kai came into Dr. Cass's office for a follow-up visit, he was almost unrecognizable. This exuberant and healthy-looking twenty-three-year-old man was very different from the moody, isolated, beer-swilling, and pot-smoking client who had come to the office months earlier. He had been given a prescription: 500 mg of each of the following—DL-phenylalanine, tyrosine, and glutamine—taken twice daily; a high vitamin B multivitamin-mineral formula, and 200–400 mg daily of Siberian ginseng. In addition, he was given 200 mcg twice daily of chromium to balance his blood sugar, and 75 mg of kava two to three times daily to reduce anxiety and help with sleep. After a month or so on the prescribed supplements, Kao's mind was calm, his mood and energy were elevated, and his addictions were curbed. Even after two later visits, he appeared to be doing quite well.

Once on the road to his personal "natural high," Kai began to search for further improvements. Soon he had discovered his own way of getting high: a meditation technique that he learned shortly after his last office visit. Not only was Kai meditating daily, but he had also managed to incorporate the new principles into his daily life.

For example, Kai recounted his preparations before going to a reggae concert with his buddies (yes, he now had friends). They were all smoking dope to put themselves in the mood for the concert. Kai described his approach:

> I just sat quietly, closed my eyes, looked upward, and soon was in a state of bliss. I was high all the way there, and during the whole show. I didn't have those old problems with coming down, either. You know—the low blood sugar and feeling bad. I can make my own high, and it's even a better one. It's free and legal, too!

Kai was rightly proud of his accomplishment, and his transformation was remarkable. Just like Kai, you, too, can produce your own natural high. The following chapters will offer several different ways to activate your own neurotransmitters—from having a positive attitude to breathing techniques, meditation, exercise, and music. Many of these techniques can help you to experience life in the present moment or, in the words of Ram Dass, to "Be here now." Much of what ails us and prevents us from attaining happiness is either remaining stuck in the past or racing toward the future. But when you recognize that the past is history—something now behind you—and that the future is a mystery waiting to unfold, then you realize that the only time that *really* exists is the present. The present is a gift (that's why it's called the present), and when you live in the present, then you're on the right track for staying high naturally.

Present and Relaxed

While most of us have to relearn the skill of living in the moment, babies and young children manage to do so effortlessly. In fact, so does your cat. Cats and babies don't worry about paying the rent, getting to the dentist on time (or the vet, for that matter), or staying in relationships. They are just there (or "here"). Is it possible for us to achieve this state? Yes, we can actually do it at a traffic light, standing in line at the bank, or waiting for a lunch date to arrive. You can turn impatience into presence. Use a breathing technique, a meditation as Kai did, or listen to specific music. There are many ways described in the following chapters that can help you find your way back to the present moment.

An integral part of being present is relaxation. This is not the sloppy relaxation of flopping in front of the TV, but relaxation as a release of tension that is often accompanied by a conscious awareness. There are many ways to relax in this way, and our individual preferences can be quite unique and personal.

One friend Lori, for example, tried using neurofeedback training (see page 239) to achieve a state of relaxed alertness, but to no avail. Session after session she simply fell asleep in the chair! In frustration, Lori decided to see what would happen if she moved around while hooked up to the device. To her surprise, the waves she produced were perfect—exactly what she had been striving for. She then recalled that when she was younger, that is exactly what she would do to get high—various forms of dance and movement. Her experience with the feedback device just proved what she had known intuitively all along.

So, there is no virtue to being an expert at *sitting* meditation if what your brain and body prefer is *movement* meditation, and vice versa. And remember, you are the best judge of what is right for you. This can also change at different periods of your life, or even from day to day.

Going with the Flow

Most of the techniques we deal with in the upcoming chapters are practices that we undertake separately from our workday lives. Whether engaged in meditation or massage, we are taking a break from our "normal" lives. Wouldn't it be great to just live that way all the time? In fact, many of us experience moments now and then in the middle of a normal day where we are absolutely in the flow. Present, unself-conscious, and focused. We often see this in dancers, rock climbers, or athletes—when they are "in the zone." Mihaly Csikszentmihalyi (pronounced chick-sent-mi-hai), the author of *Flow: The Psychology of Optimal Experience,* has pursued for years the question of how we might experience this more often. He has found that certain conditions are conducive to our finding flow—when we are actively involved in a difficult enterprise that stretches our physical or mental abilities, when challenges are high, and when our personal skills are used to the utmost.

The first sign of flow is a narrowing of attention on a clearly defined goal—we know what must be done. If we can get consistent feedback as to how well we're doing, even a boring job can become exciting and engaging. For flow to occur, we need to experience clear goals, immediate feedback, and a dynamic tension between challenges and skills. Once the challenges are brought into balance with our skills and the goals are clarified, we can slip into this magical timeless space of flow, one of the best natural highs there is.

Fun and Laughter

Don't forget, too, that play and laughter are still two of the all-time best ways to get high: a good belly laugh gets your muscles relaxed, your oxygen flowing, your neurotransmitters firing, and your immune system enhanced. And, while you're laughing, you can't help but be in the moment.

Here are some other simple ways to get yourself into the "here and now":

- Take a deep breath, let it go, and as you slowly exhale fully, come back to yourself. Repeat this several times. Instead of worrying about what is not happening, allow yourself to be exactly where you are. You'll find that time will shift, then stand still, and you will feel alive, connected, and energized.
- Take a quiet walk. Try the beach, a park, or any special place where you can let go of your worries. Enjoy a beautiful sunset. Nature can be the best "awakener"—as we sink into her rhythm, we discover that ultimately it is also our own. Even reminiscing about a pleasant experience from the past will bring us into a happier connection with "now," as our bodies recall the good feelings of "then."
- Try a more structured form of relaxation therapy if it suits you. Exercise, movement, breathing exercises, yoga, meditation, biofeedback, self-hypnosis, and t'ai chi all are techniques that can help you to approach life with a greater sense of inner calm and expansiveness. With many of these, it takes only 10 to 15 minutes a day to see results. It often helps to do these techniques in a group. Aside from the fun of social contact, the group energy seems to prime the pump, making it easier to reach a relaxed, altered state.

In each of the following chapters, we will describe an activity, how it helps to produce a natural high, and will provide a simple exercise for you to try. You will soon see that the common theme running throughout is the state of being fully aware and in the present. Allow all of your senses to come into play—sight, sound, taste, touch, movement—whether you are meditating, deep breathing, exercising, dancing, listening to music, inhaling aromatic oils, massaging or being massaged, or making love. Enjoy them! These exercises are all free, legal, and safe.

11

Moving Toward Bliss

Remember how you felt as a child, running and playing with your whole being—body, mind, and spirit? We adults can still recapture some of that same high with a variety of activities. And they don't have to be the stereotype of ".exercise," which often conjures up images of regimentation, discomfort, and even punishment! Something as simple as a hike in the hills can leave you feeling exhilarated and at one with the world around you.

We are already aware of the many physical benefits of exercise: controlling weight, toning muscles, strengthening bones, conditioning the heart and lungs, and maintaining flexibility in our joints. But aerobic exercise can also improve our moods by producing positive changes in our bodies and brain chemistries. Aerobic exercise not only reduces the release of adrenal stress hormones but also increases the supply of blood and oxygen to the brain, enhancing memory. Exercise stimulates the growth of new brain cells in the hippocampus, the area responsible for memory. In a study published in 1999, Professor Arthur Beckman at the University of Illinois tested 124 adults over a six-month period. Half the group did three 45-minute walks a week, while the other half did stretching and toning. The aerobic group had a 15 to 20 percent improvement in short-term memory, recall, and response time, while the other group showed no improvement. Of course, this is not to say that stretching and toning are not beneficial.

Endorphins and Mood Enhancement

Exercise also stimulates the release of powerful, mood-elevating endorphins. These chemical messengers can create a state of euphoria and relieve pain, with effects that are often hundreds of times stronger than those produced by morphine. This natural "opium" produces the addictive sensation commonly known as "runner's high." Deprived of their "fix," grounded runners will often become irritable and depressed, acting much like addicts deprived of their drugs.

There have been more than one hundred clinical studies examining the link between endorphins and exercise. One of the most interesting was conducted by Dr. Dennis Lobstein at the University of New Mexico. He compared ten sedentary men with ten of similar age who jogged. He discovered that the sedentary men were more depressed and had lower levels of endorphins, along with higher levels of stress hormones, than the joggers. Not surprisingly, the sedentary subjects also perceived higher levels of stress in their lives. Other studies have since established that exercise can be as effective as antidepressants or traditional psychotherapy for treating low moods, possibly due to its effects in raising endorphin levels.

In another experiment, investigators found that aerobic exercise can elevate the body's levels of phenylethylamine (PEA), a natural chemical— part of the endorphin-induced "runner's high"—that enhances energy, mood, and attention. When researchers had twenty healthy young men run on a treadmill for 30 minutes, they found that the average concentration of PEA in the participants' urine increased by 77 percent. In addition, the report indicated that patients suffering from depression and bipolar disorder had lower-than-normal levels of PEA in their urine.

However, you don't have to be either depressed or a seasoned athlete to benefit from exercise. The more intensely you exercise, the more of these chemicals you produce, and the higher you get. Exercise can also increase self-esteem, as tangible evidence of your desire to take charge of your life.

Here is a testimonial, from Oliver, a forty-three-year-old musician:

> *I used to be into all kinds of stimulants, including cocaine. Since I discovered running, I have a clear and consistent high. I feel terrific most of the time, without the lows I used to have after coke. I would not trade this feeling for anything.*

Unlocking Vital Energy

Scientific research has found that yoga and t'ai chi produce additional health benefits. T'ai chi can boost well-being and immunity, while yoga has been shown to have positive effects on pulse, blood pressure, and mental and physical performance—benefits that are beyond those seen from physical exercise alone.

By unblocking the flow of vital energy, known in China as *chi* and in India as *prana,* you can restore your vitality, returning to a natural and blissful state of equilibrium.

YOGA: STRENGTH, EQUILIBRIUM, AND VITALITY

Practicing yoga can provide relaxation, clarity of mind, and increased energy. The word *yoga* comes from the Sanskrit word for "union." Its origins can be traced back over thousands of years to the very foundation of Indian civilization. In its truest form, yoga is the science and practice of obtaining freedom and liberation. The physical exercises of hatha yoga are only one type of the discipline, in which breath, movement, and posture are harmonized to remove physical blocks and tension in the body. As emotional tension is also stored in the body, the aim of hatha yoga is to promote physical, emotional, mental, *and* spiritual well-being.

Hatha yoga has many styles, such as Iyengar yoga, which is a slower and more precise form. It uses a series of postures to help realign the body to enhance the flow of vital energy. Astanga yoga, on the other hand, is a more athletic and physically demanding type of yoga. Both forms will leave you feeling more relaxed and energized. Try them both and see what suits you.

Yoga classes are now widely available and a great path to a natural high. Simon was vice-president of a record company, with a very busy life and a lot of stress. He tried many alternative approaches, but it was yoga that made the biggest difference. Simon explains:

> When I started doing yoga, I experienced a sustained energy release that lasted all day. I got into a routine of doing a yoga session almost every day. As well as giving me more energy, I feel much more positive, and how I react to stress has changed. Things that used to bother me before don't cause me anywhere near the same degree of agitation. Practicing yoga hasn't made me slow down, either. I'm still very busy but I'm much calmer about everything.

Simon found the benefits of yoga so great that he now teaches at the Triyoga Center in London!

Once you've learned the postures, you can practice yoga at home, perhaps accompanied by an instruction video or some relaxing music.

T'AI CHI: MEDITATION IN MOTION

T'ai chi chuan is another vitality-generating physical exercise. Originating in China, its aim is to allow the *chi*, or vital energy, to flow unhindered throughout the body. T'ai chi involves learning a series of precise movements that flow into each other. They are a form of martial arts and are like shadow-boxing in slow motion.

The fluid movements of t'ai chi help you learn how to relax certain muscles, rather than tensing them, and help to reduce the level of background tension that we all hold within our bodies. These movements also open up the joints to allow our *chi* to flow unhindered. T'ai chi therefore helps to develop harmony with the self through posture and strength through yielding. Once the sequence is learned through attending classes with a qualified teacher, t'ai chi can be practiced at home.

You'll feel more connected and alert when you practice t'ai chi, with an inner calm. Robert, age sixty-six, took up t'ai chi when he retired. Here's how he describes the benefits:

> *I've never been an athletic person or good at anything physical. T'ai chi, however, I enjoy immensely. I like the feeling of being "in control" of my body. I do it almost every day for 20 minutes. It increases my energy and clears my mind. It gives me a kind of equilibrium that has many benefits, such as helping me to play my violin better and helping me to stay detached when things are bad. I find it very calming when I'm stressed or upset.*

PSYCHOCALISTHENICS: AEROBIC YOGA?

Psychocalisthenics is the brainchild of Oscar Ichazo, founder of the Arica School for the understanding of the complete person. A practitioner of marital arts and yoga since 1939, he has developed a routine of twenty-three exercises that can be done in less than 20 minutes. A complete contemporary exercise system that looks like a powerful form of aerobic yoga, Psychocalisthenics is designed to become "a serious foundation for a life of self-responsibility, clarity of mind, and strength of spirit," according to Ichazo. It generates both physical fitness and vital energy by bringing mind and body into balance, a key being the precise breathing pattern that accompanies each physical exercise.

When we first started doing this unique routine of movement, breath, and exercises, we were amazed at how light, reenergized, and "high" we felt afterward. Other advocates of Psychocalisthenics give the same glowing reports: "This is exercise pared to perfection. I wasn't sweating buckets as I would after an aerobics class, but I could feel I had exercised far more muscles. I was feeling clear-headed and bright rather than wiped out," said Jane Alexander, in a *Daily Mail* review. Once you've learned the routine, you can do it in under 20 minutes in your own home, accompanied either by the video- or audiotape. (See Resources.)

Natural Highs

INVITATION TO THE DANCE

Dancing to music is one of the most powerful (and primal) ways to release endorphins. One of the pioneers of dance as a natural high is Gabrielle Roth, who writes, "I feel my soul in my body when I dance." She describes the night she discovered this:

> *I got up and started moving, holding nothing back, nothing at all. Lost in the spirit of the dance, I found a path, a dancing path, that took me to the deepest most alive place I had ever seen. . . . It was as if I were plugged into the master current and life was charging through me, creating a clarity that I had never known before.*

Her talented and soulful musicians will make you dance to your depths, like there is no tomorrow. Sweat a little—it's good for you. You won't be able to stop smiling. Notice variations in mood and tempo, from flowing to staccato, and from chaos to lyrical, as you explore your body and soul in motion. Dance 20 minutes a day, and you will be reconnected with yourself. This form of exercise is also a form of moving meditation, so why not combine the two?

GROUNDING BEFORE FLYING

. . . we need only to disappear in the dance to liberate the sexual, creative, and sacred aspects of the soul . . . Energy moves in waves. Waves move in patterns. Patterns move in rhythms. A human being is just that, energy, waves, patterns, rhythms. Nothing more. Nothing less. A dance.
GABRIELLE ROTH, *SWEAT YOUR PRAYERS*

Just like the rest of nature—rivers, trees, clouds, and stars—we are in constant inner movement. Our organs, muscles, nerves, and body fluids dance in ever-unfolding patterns. Emilie Conrad Da'oud has been teaching this for years in her famous "Continuum" class. She demonstrates how the tiniest movements can resonate throughout the body—how the slightest twitch of a finger can be as powerful as a full-body leap. Try it: you will find your whole body very subtly vibrating. We can refer to quantum physics for validation of this phenomenon: all life is vibration.

Dr. Joanne Segel, a pioneer in movement research and therapy, notes that, as we become fully and vitally aware of these subtle inner patterns— of the living structures within us—we are better able to *embody* ourselves. She emphasizes the importance of going on to *ground* yourself in this body awareness—"We can go as high as we go deep." That is, we must first connect with our bodies and the earth beneath us before we can transcend and fly. A trained dancer who wants to leap high into the air first imagines *sinking down* into the floor or even into the earth below. She bends her knees and sends her energy down, grounding herself, connecting with her support, *before soaring into space.* A great analogy for all of us: feel your center and your support, before you leap beyond it.

It seems, then, that vitality, the very real experience of feeling naturally high, is more than just the consequence of your diet, physical fitness, and state of mind. The extra factor is the one that's hardest to measure but no less tangible. Vital energy is sometimes described as the energy we draw in from the universe, and, depending on how receptive we are, it has the power to nourish us at a fundamental level. All the disciplines we've discussed above are designed to make us more receptive. So, too, is acupuncture, which works by unblocking channels of energy, called *meridians,* through which this vital energy is said to flow. When you walk by the ocean, lie on a beach, or walk in the woods on a sunny day, you feel more "connected," more "in touch," with a perspective on life far removed from the one you have, say, when commuting to work. Vital energy is that hidden ingredient that connects us with one another and with the world around us, allowing us to feel at one with it all.

Vital Energy Enhancers

- Whatever form of exercise you choose, it's easier if you do it with a friend. Besides providing company and being more fun, this partnering keeps you committed.
- If you have never exercised before, and especially if you have a pre-existing health condition, see your doctor before you begin.
- Start your exercise program gradually, with something as simple as a walk around the block.
- Build up over time to a slow jog around the neighborhood or on a track, slowly increasing the distance and speed.
- For maximum benefit, build up to a full jog that lasts between 20 and 30 minutes, four to six days a week.
- Jogging, cycling, swimming, and calisthenics all are forms of *aerobic exercise,* which conditions the heart and lungs. So is dancing, as mentioned earlier.
- Weight lifting provides *resistance exercise,* which both builds muscles and counters osteoporosis, since bone development is stimulated by weight-bearing exercise. It also helps to burn fat. Both types of exercise are important to overall health.
- All exercise takes your mind off your worries: think of the times when you played tag, baseball, or basketball with your friends. Be a kid again!
- Ride your bike, in-line skate, or use an exercise bike while watching a video or reading a book.
- Practice yoga, t'ai chi, or Psychocalisthenics in a class or with video instruction at least twice a week, if not daily. Class instruction will teach the correct movements, and the group setting can inspire and energize.
- Turn on your favorite music and dance—a form of moving meditation. Do this 20 minutes a day, and you will be reconnected with yourself.
- If you get moving five days a week, you will feel fabulous and look great, too. Whatever activities you choose, keep the following tips in mind:

- Wear loose, comfortable clothing and well-fitting shoes, appropriate to the activity.
- Warm up before exercise, stretch muscles before and after, and perform cool-down exercises.
- Do not fall into the "no pain, no gain" trap. Some muscular soreness or tightness is normal, especially if these activities are new, but pain is a sign that something is wrong. If the pain persists, stop exercising and see your health-care practitioner.
- Don't overdo it, especially at the beginning. Give yourself a day off between exercise sessions. Excessive exercise actually evokes the stress response.
- Do something you enjoy. The more you enjoy an exercise, the more likely you are to stick with it.

12

The Breath of Life

Breathing is something we take for granted. Yet it is no accident that the earliest meanings of the word *inspire* include "to breathe life into." Over the centuries, it has come to mean "to fill with enlivening or exalting emotion," "to stimulate to action," "to stimulate energies, ideals, or reverence," and, finally, "to affect, guide, or arouse by divine influence." In fact, the word for breath and for spirit were once the same, meaning "the vital principle or animating force within living beings." This is reflected in the Hebrew word for *breath*—"ruach"—which means "the spirit."

For thousands of years in India, people have practiced breathing exercises called *pranayama* that are designed to help one attain good health, high energy, and a blissful state of mind. In the next chapter, we will describe the use of the breath in meditation and during exercise. In this chapter, we cover some basic techniques and explain how proper breathing benefits health, relaxation, and energy levels.

Breath and Emotion

Your breathing is a reflection of your emotions: when you are anxious or afraid, the stress response causes your breathing to become rapid and shallow. When you are happy and at ease, your breathing becomes slow and deep. It works both ways, too. You can use how you breathe to calm an agitated mind and tense body.

You can try this yourself right now. Bring to mind something you are stressed or anxious about. Put it to one side for a minute, and focus on your breath. Let your inhalation become a little deeper and your exhalation a little longer with each breath. Take several slow breaths like this, and notice how "detached" you become from the emotional charge, with a new perspective on your situation. You can see why conscious breathing is a fundamental part of meditation and yoga and is vital to any natural relaxation program.

Oxygenate Your Body

Oxygen may be the most important nutrient of all. You can live thirty days without food and four days without water, but cut off from oxygen, you will die in only four minutes. We often assume that we all get enough oxygen from breathing, but, in fact, our oxygen supply is dependent on both the depth of our breathing and the quality of air we breathe. Compare how you feel when breathing refreshing mountain air with trying *not* to inhale the smoggy city air.

As oxygen travels throughout the body, it is taken up into cells—in exchange for carbon dioxide—to produce cellular energy. When we don't get a sufficient supply of oxygen, we feel tired, cranky, and dull due to an increase in carbon dioxide levels. Then, after taking a few really deep breaths, our cells become recharged with fresh oxygen and life goes from a dull gray to a bright technicolor. For those of us who have never breathed fully and well, this experience can be a revelation.

Optimal health and wellness are impossible without optimal breathing. This may seem self-evident, but most of us breathe shallowly—just enough to get by. To give yourself a natural energy boost and keep yourself relaxed and clearheaded, stay conscious of your breath. Breathe fully and deeply. Also, avoid places that have poor or stagnant air, such as smoke-filled bars.

Physical exercise and breathing exercises will help you to maximize your lung capacity. Most of us use less than one-third of it! The best ways to oxygenate your tissues, improving energy and alertness, are aerobic, stamina-building exercises such as swimming, jogging, cycling, and brisk walking. They all require that you breathe deeper and harder. When you exercise, synchronize your movements with your breath. This will help you to breathe deeply, producing a natural oxygen high, with energy, exhilaration, and a natural connection. Your mind and body become "in sync." We also have some exercises that you can try: Dia-Kath breathing, progressive relaxation, and vibrance breathing.

DIAKATH BREATHING

This breathing exercise (reproduced with the kind permission of the Arica Institute, a school for self-knowledge) connects the *kath* point—the body's center of equilibrium—with the diaphragm muscle so that deep breathing becomes natural and effortless. You can practice this exercise at any time, while sitting, standing, or lying down, and for as long as you like. You can also do it unobtrusively during moments of stress. It is an excellent natural relaxant and energy booster, helping you to feel more connected and in tune.

The diaphragm is a dome-shaped muscle attached to the bottom of the rib cage. The *kath* is not an anatomical point like the navel but is located in the lower belly, about three finger-widths below the navel. When you remember this point, you become aware of your entire body.

In Diakath breathing, your lower belly expands from the *kath* point as you inhale. The diaphragm muscle expands downward as if pulled by the *kath* point. This allows the lungs to fill with air from the bottom to the top. As you exhale, the belly and the diaphragm muscle relax, allowing the lungs to empty from top to bottom. Inhale and exhale through your nose.

Diakath Breathing: Step by Step

1. Sit comfortably, in a quiet place with your spine straight.
2. Focus your attention on your *kath* point.
3. Let your belly expand from the *kath* point as you inhale slowly, deeply, and effortlessly. Feel your diaphragm being pulled down toward the *kath* point as your lungs fill with air from the bottom to the top. On the exhale, relax both your belly and your diaphragm, emptying your lungs from top to bottom.
4. Repeat at your own pace.

Every morning sit down in a quiet place before breakfast and practice Diakath breathing for a few minutes. Breathing this way can lead you into meditation. Whenever you are stressed throughout the day, check your breathing. Practice Diakath breathing for nine breaths. This is great to do before an important meeting or when something has upset you.

Diakath Breathing™ and Kath™ are trademarks of Oscar Ichazo. Used by permission.

PROGRESSIVE RELAXATION

When you feel the need to de-stress and unwind, try this breathing exercise called progressive relaxation. First, lie down and take several deep, slow breaths. Then, breathe in slowly as you tense the muscles in your foot. Hold your breath and maintain the tension in your foot for a count of twenty. (If you don't make it to twenty at the beginning, don't worry.) After counting to twenty, slowly exhale, releasing your muscles until they are totally relaxed. Repeat this process next with your calf muscles, then the thigh, buttocks, and so on, slowly working your way up to finish with your facial muscles. Close with a few more deep breaths.

BREATHING FOR VIBRANCE

International seminar leader and author Gay Hendricks has explored the subject of breathing for many years. The result is a powerful series of vibrance techniques, shared below. You can find out more in his book *Achieving Vibrance,* and on his Web site (www.hendricks.com).

There are three specific errors that the majority of people make in their breathing, which Hendricks calls "The Central Breathing Problem":

- breathing too shallowly.
- breathing too fast.
- breathing "upside down."

The obvious solution is to breathe more slowly, deeply, and right side up. Upside-down breathing doesn't mean we breathe standing on our heads! Read on and you'll understand what it is.

The best way to understand healthy breathing is to watch a baby breathe. When a baby inhales, its belly rises and rounds. The belly muscles stay relaxed, so that the breath can get deep down into the bottom of his lungs. When you see an unhealthy adult breathe, the exact opposite occurs (which is why it's called upside-down breathing).

Most adults hold their belly muscles too tightly, which keeps the lungs from expanding fully. Imagine wearing a tight girdle around your middle. When your breath comes in, the expansion of your lungs comes up against this immovable wall. Since the belly can't relax and round, the lungs cannot expand to their fullest. Something has to give. What happens is that the "girdle around the middle" causes the breath to be forced up into the chest, inflating it to accommodate the pressure. When you breathe high in your chest, you must take short, shallow breaths at a faster rate, as opposed to the slower, deeper breathing that occurs when you keep your belly relaxed.

You feel several specific sensations when your "breathing chemistry" is out of balance:

- Tired all the time, even when you first wake up.
- Anxious, even though you may not be able to point to anything disturbing in your environment.
- Unable to get a full breath.
- Lost in a mental fog.

The Central Breathing Problem can usually be remedied fairly quickly. Most people can get the basics in under an hour by following simple self-help instructions. The moment you get your breathing balanced, you will feel an immediate sense of ease and an enhanced state of well-being. You'll learn how below.

The Vibrance-Breath: Beginning Instructions

Begin by sitting comfortably upright. First, let's review how to breathe in coordination with the natural way your spine is designed to move. When you were a baby, your spine and breathing were naturally coordinated. Later, as the stresses of living caused tension in your body, your breathing may have gone out of harmony with the flexing of your spine.

So we begin this exercise with spinal movement. First arch and flatten the small of your back gently, taking 3 to 4 seconds to arch and 3 to 4 seconds to flatten. As you arch the small of your back, look toward the ceiling, and when you flatten the small of your back, look toward the floor. Don't strain your neck when you look up or down—just a few inches of movement will do just fine. Do a few cycles of this movement until it feels easy and natural.

Now, begin to breathe in harmony with your spinal movement. Breathe in as you arch the small of your back, and breathe out as you flatten the small of your back. Relax your stomach muscles so your belly can round as you breathe in. Continue to look up when you breathe in and look down when you breathe out. Keep the same easy rhythm—3 to 4 seconds to breathe in and 3 to 4 seconds to breathe out. Repeat this for a few cycles, keeping it gentle and easy.

The Vibrance-Breath During the Day

Hendricks notes that, even though he has felt balanced and harmonious for many years, he still practices for a few minutes every morning: "I think of it as a bit of fine-tuning to help my body remember what the sensations of balance feel like." You can also do the Vibrance-Breath during the day if you get jangled, fatigued, or foggy. Practice at your desk or as you walk around. You can even do a subtle form of the activity in public—riding in cabs, giving speeches, in lines, or during meetings. Once you learn it, you'll have a friend for life.

13

Meditation and the Mind

Prayer is like talking to God, meditation is a way of listening to God.
EDGAR CAYCE

M editation is one of the best natural highs of all. It helps promote mental clarity and a sense of connection and will simultaneously increase your energy, improve your mood, and keep you calm. While most of us have become familiar with meditation through Eastern religions, Judaism, Islam, and Christianity have their meditation traditions as well. In fact, most of the world's religions have meditation as a central devotional activity in their quest for connection with the Divine. Aside from the spiritual component, meditation has a multitude of benefits for the mind and body.

Not only is it great for your state of mind, it also has many positive benefits for your body, including better responsiveness to stressful events and quicker recovery, reduced heart rate and blood pressure, a slowed rate of breathing, and more stable brain-wave patterns.

Meditation has also been shown to prevent the depression of the body's immune responses that occurs with stress. People who practice meditation on a regular basis have been found to be less anxious, and there is little doubt that meditation and relaxation techniques are effective in dealing with anxiety, stress, and insomnia. This confirms research at the University of Massachusetts Medical Center that found that meditators have lower levels of the stress hormone cortisol.

In Chapter 4 we have seen how even the mildest conflicts can generate an exaggerated "fight or flight" stress reaction (more appropriately reserved for dealing with life-threatening situations). Meditation can be the way to help us unlearn this conditioned response and become less reactive to the normal stresses and strains of life.

How do you bring about this state of balance? Most meditation techniques involve focusing on one object, such as the breath or a mantra (a sound, such as "om"), for a period of time—say, 10 to 20 minutes—and on a regular basis. Ordinarily, the brain and body are bombarded with a multitude of signals, such as thought processes (mental), hunger (physical), or fear (emotional). This can lead to overstimulation, with resulting confusion, encumberance, and stress. On the other hand, by focusing on the breath, as we saw in the previous chapter, or a sound such as "om," we are letting go of the stimuli as soon as they are perceived. This peaceful result is diametrically opposed to the modern experience of stress and exhaustion with the mind darting from one problem to another, leaving a trail of panic.

With practice, the power of the mind seems to grow, and, with that, your mental concentration and energy improve. With regular meditation, the mind becomes quieter. You learn to focus on the important tasks at hand, rather than dissipating your energy by trying (unsuccessfully) to do many things at once. However, even this benefit is superficial when compared with what happens at deeper levels of meditation. This is how co-author Patrick Holford experienced one deep meditation:

I had a firsthand experience of this during a two-day siddha yoga meditation weekend intensive. The highlight for me was on the second day when the meditation master gave a fascinating talk explaining all about the nature of the mind and how we can lose touch with the inner self. By this time, not being very good at sitting on the floor, my body was aching and my mind was tired and bursting at the seams.

Then she led us into meditation by chanting "om." As I did this, the sound "om" began reverberating inside me as if my body were a vast, empty cave. The sound reverberated outside me, filling the hall as if it were a magnificent cathedral. It was an extraordinary and very uplifting sensation.

Suddenly, the chanting stopped. There was not a sound. Everything went black. My mind literally stopped thinking. My body stopped aching. In fact, it felt so blissful that not a single muscle stirred. There was just this delicious, empty silence. Occasionally a thought would come up like a ship on the horizon and then pass from view. I felt no emotion as such, just this pure, deep, total contentment. Every moment and every breath was so exquisite. I just sat there observing every millimeter of every breath come in, and go out, like the waves on the beach. When I opened my eyes, the hall was empty and all the people had gone and I realized an hour had passed.

Since then, meditation has been like dipping into a well of rejuvenating tranquility. It has given me a place inside where I can see everything from a clearer perspective.

How Meditation Integrates Your Brain

With time and good instruction, those who meditate find they can slip into an elevated state of awareness—a kind of pure "being"—in which the mind becomes naturally still, the body relaxes, and all emotions settle. This state is real—not imagined—and correlates to distinctive changes in brain-wave patterns that shift from the high-activity beta waves that predominate in our awake state, to a slower alpha wave rhythm, and finally into theta wave activity. In Chapter 14, we describe how you can actually train your brain waves to achieve this state with neurofeedback.

James Thornton, director of the Heffter Research Institute for exploring new frontiers in neuroscience and consciousness, explains how focus on the breath helps bring the brain into balance:

Breathing is controlled by the oldest brain: the reptilian brain. The awareness [of the breath] is actually in the new brain, the neocortex. You integrate the experience of your brain by focusing the awareness in the big new human brain on the activities of the old small reptile brain and at that point, you've got a fully integrated brain functioning.

Oscar Ichazo, who invented psychocalisthenics, is also a modern-day master of meditation. He says:

They mystical experience happens to us when and only when our cortex becomes unified or harmonized in such a way that it immediately starts working on a different level. Our mind starts going to the

Meditation Exercise

1. Sit in a quiet place and adopt a comfortable posture with your spine straight. If you are sitting cross-legged on the floor, you may find it helpful to straighten your spine by tucking a firm cushion under your pelvis.
2. Let go of any tension in your body and feel your spine elongate.
3. Become aware of your breath and start Diakath Breathing (see page 228) for nine breaths.
4. Now let your breathing find its own rhythm. Bring your awareness to the place in your body where your breath arises. With each exhalation, bring your awareness to the place to where your breath goes.
5. Whenever your mind wanders, bring it back to the breath. There is no need to resist your thoughts as such—simply become aware that your focus has shifted to your thoughts and gently bring it back to the breath.

Do this meditation exercise for at least 10 minutes daily, ideally at the beginning or end of the day. This is as refreshing as having a good night's sleep.

Whenever you are stressed, in an unpleasant mood, or are feeling disconnected, practice meditation by sitting quietly for 5 or more minutes. If you would like to deepen your experience of meditation, see Resources for details on meditation courses.

lowest vibrations of the EEG scale (which is a measure of the quality of brain activity). Everyone agrees that the state of meditation is produced by the alpha wave. But if we descend to the theta wave we can produce even higher states. That is when all the activities of the cerebral cortex have been pacified in a way that then it is one unity and one solid experience of our entire being. In every mystical tradition the teaching is precisely to train people to the point where they can reproduce in themselves this state of totality of the cerebral cortex.

To reach this level of expertise in meditation it certainly helps to follow the instruction of a meditation master. In time, and with practice, meditation can help you experience an increase in your energy, mental clarity, and ability to stay unaffected by the turbulence of daily life—and, just possibly, awaken you to that "bigger picture" in which everything in life falls into place. Instead of being blindly limited to viewing life as "a struggle" or "survival of the fittest," we can awaken to the oneness, the connectedness, the play of life. This is the true goal of meditation and the ultimate natural high.

14

Biofeedback, Relaxation, and the Alpha State

Did you know that you have the ability to voluntarily alter your pulse, blood pressure, and even your brain waves? For many years, scientists assumed that we couldn't affect our so-called "autonomic" functions. Then Western researchers discovered yogis who could stop and start their hearts at will. Later Tibetan monks—seemingly able to generate endless amounts of energy—were found capable of melting huge quantities of ice with their bodies. If any of us tried it, our bodies would become so cold we'd die, but these monks didn't appear to be adversely affected. And just as these highly trained people can influence their physiology and mental states, scientists have developed powerful biofeedback technology that allows us to perform similar feats.

There are many ways to get into an alpha state. Many people study meditation, learn yoga, listen to specific music, or practice exercises, such as those suggested in Dr. Herbert Benson's landmark book *The Relaxation Response*. Another technique made famous by Dr. John Lilly involves flotation in an isolation tank—a process that induces a deep alpha state that has been known to create profound shifts after as little as one session.

Neurofeedback: Tame the Mind

The most direct form of biofeedback for altering your mental state is neurofeedback. Neurofeedback helps to tame the restless mind while promoting relaxation and balance on all levels—mental, emotional, physical, and spiritual. The key here is the alpha brain-wave state, a true resting place where the brain and body recover from stress.

Sensing electrodes are attached to various parts of the scalp, connecting the user to an electroencephalogram (EEG), a computer that detects brain-wave patterns. These brain rhythms can then be observed on a computer screen. By seeing how changes in your internal state can affect your brain-wave patterns, you can learn how to shift them by training your mind to move into different states, ranging from focused attention to deep relaxation.

In a deeply relaxed, meditative state, your physical body produces a vibration that measures at about 8 cycles per second (cps). At the same time, your brain waves shift from their everyday waking beta range (13–39 cps) into the same 8 cps deep alpha range as the body. When this occurs, an electromagnetic field is created around the head. Amazingly, this field links up with the frequency of the earth's electromagnetic field, hovering around 8 cycles per second. Then, once we are in harmony with the planetary vibration, we feel high!

One of the leading pioneers in biofeedback techniques is Dr. Les Fehmi, whose early research experience is described in Jim Robbins's book *Symphony in the Brain: The Evolution of the New Brain Wave Biofeedback*. Visit www.symphonyinthebrain.com for more information. This excerpt will give you a good idea of how it works:

> *After weeks of frustration, going nowhere, Dr. Les Fehmi once more hooked himself up to the EEG monitor. Instead of concentrating hard and focusing intently on his goal, however, this time he relaxed his focus and let go. Much to his surprise, profound feelings washed over him, and then, his life began to change dramatically. He felt far more relaxed and at ease in his body, and he adopted a more*

centered attitude toward life. Physical changes happened as well. Severe, long-term arthritis in his hands disappeared, and his vision and sense of smell were enhanced. He knew that this was the way life was meant to be!

Dr. Fehmi continued working with himself and many others over the years and came to the conclusion that a fundamental problem in our culture is that we are taught as children to focus too narrowly on the external world. With our minds and eyes, we literally grip objects and the outside world too intently. This leads to problems such as anxiety and depression. Fehmi now coaches people in methods to relax their grip. As they learn to do that, the rest of the body's physiology relaxes as well.

In case you are wondering, you don't have to be wired up to an EEG monitor to benefit from Dr. Fehmi's biofeedback research. He has developed a set of audiotapes that help you to move quickly into the desired state. Robbins describes his own experience using these tapes, feeling lighter, happier, and more energetic. His senses were also enhanced: "I could pick up the smell of lilacs blooming half a block away. The sun seemed more golden, richer somehow, the way I remembered it glowing from childhood." Visit www.openfocus.com for more information.

The secret to achieving an alpha state in neurofeedback (as in any meditative practice) as Dr. Fehmi disovered is being present in the moment and letting go into expanded awareness. Along similar lines, Dr. James Hardt describes how hundreds of people have had profound spiritual experiences during the course of his Biocybernaut EEG Training, often with life-transforming results. Visit www.biocybernaut.com for more information.

Mind Mirror

Anna Wise, a leading teacher in the field of biofeedback, utilizes the Mind Mirror, a neurofeedback device originally developed in England by Max Cade, and further refined by Wise. Encouraging optimal performance as well as spiritual connection, the Mind Mirror helps you access your various mind states, which can be seen as wave patterns on a computer screen. Through training, you learn to create any state you desire: alpha for deep relaxation, beta for focused thought, theta for creative inspiration, and delta for restful sleep. When the various rhythms are in harmony and balance, a specific wave form shows up on the monitor.

Whether or not you own a Mind Mirror (and you can!), you can learn to access, maximize, and harmonize your various mind states with the help of Anna Wise's books and CDs. Visit www.annawise.com for more information.

VibraSound

Developed by Don Estes—a brilliant scientist, inventor, and author— VibraSound Total Sensory Wave Table is an innovative device for changing brain frequency. VibraSound uses biosensors to measure your personal sound vibration. This is then analyzed by a complex computer program to produce your unique "sound fingerprint," called the spectral absorption signature (SAS). Like your fingerprint, your SAS is stable and reproducible, regardless of how you are feeling at the time. The VibraSound then feeds back to your body the exact sounds, colors, and vibrotactile information needed to harmonize and balance your "vibration." All you need to do is lay there and soak it in! People describe feeling blissed out for days afterward. In fact, some report lasting changes in their overall emotions and attitudes after just one session. Visit www.vibrasound.com for more information.

For a simpler approach, you can listen to a tape or CD of musicians that has been shown to induce a deep alpha state. (See Resources.) Find a peaceful and comfortable place to listen to an alpha wave–inducing tape, such as Fehmi's *Open Focus,* Anna Wise's *Awakening the Mind,* or Steven Halpern's Anti-Frantic series, for 20 minutes daily.

15

Positive Thinking

Much of our suffering is created in our own minds. We set the scene by how we react to things that stress us out, make us feel down, and zap our energy. Overly pessimistic feelings can make us even more depressed and negative. If we look deeper, often we realize that many supposedly "bad" events in life, like the end of a relationship or the loss of a job, actually turn out to be blessings, both in terms of what we learn and for the space these events create for new possibilities. Even life-threatening illness, or the tragic loss of a loved one, can be an opportunity for positive change. It's this kind of thinking that can keep us growing, moving, and happy with our lives.

Part of our evolutionary programming is to be on the lookout for external threats. We also learn this early in life through our relationships with our parents, from whom we learn ways of reacting to the world. These negative patterns are usually based on deep-seated false premises, such as "No one will love me as I am," or "I am never good enough," or "There is something wrong with me." As a result, we attract situations and gravitate toward people who fit our negative views of life—people who abandon us or criticize us, and situations in which we are destined to fail or cannot live up to other people's expectations. These patterns are so deep-seated that they are hard to see. Whenever you say to yourself or others, "You never . . ." or "You always . . ." you can be pretty certain you are seeing the situation through a deep-rooted negative pattern. These are often reflections of our parents' negative traits or attitudes. And it's not their fault, since they inherited them from *their* parents.

Breaking the Pattern

All this negativity can leave us feeling helpless, unable to express who we are or to do the things we really want to do. Instead of engaging in life and being in the moment, we feel bored, depressed, and unfulfilled. Maybe it wasn't safe for you as a child to be angry, or you were brought up being told that "boys don't cry." As a result you might say, "I'm fine," when you're actually angry or sad.

The good news is that, just as we were able to learn our negative patterns, we are also able to *unlearn* them. One of the first steps to breaking a pattern is to be truthful about how you feel. This can even be done in private—in your personal journal or in an unsent letter. Releasing unexpressed emotions can liberate a lot of energy, and you will probably find yourself feeling lighter, even high.

Once in that state of mind, you can replace the old negative image or belief with a positive one, such as I am OK; I deserve to feel good; I deserve to have what I want; I am safe and protected; or I can take care of myself. These are the positive messages we might have missed in childhood. But one of the miracles of human consciousness is that it's never too late to have a happy childhood. To the unconscious mind, time is irrelevant. You can change your inner program, heal your frightened inner child, and live a happy life. It sounds simple, but our minds are in some ways quite basic. As you think, so you are.

Start by being good to yourself. As well as doing all the things you do for others, your partner, your friends, and your children, do something for yourself. Take up a hobby or activity that you always wanted to do. Buy yourself something. Get a massage. Go for a hike. Have lunch with a friend. Go to the zoo. Do something fun, even for a short time, every day.

You can say that life isn't that kind to us, and we are always going to be faced with challenges, including huge losses. This is true. However, while we might not always realize it, we really can choose how we perceive and respond to difficult situations. Prisoners have been grateful for the beauty of the ray of sunlight that filters through a chink in the stone walls.

If we just remember that we can, we are able to change our responses to those stressful times—from mundane daily events like standing in a slow-moving bank line, cramming for a final exam, or responding to a demanding two-year-old, to the larger, life- or health-threatening possibilities that loom over us.

It pays to be up! Optimism and a positive attitude go a long way toward helping us maintain good health. Research shows that the higher your optimism, the healthier your immune system. Moreover, the likelier it is that good things will happen to you. Negative expectations actually breed negative experiences. It sometimes takes work to be happy, not allowing yourself to give in to self-pity.

The HeartMath® Solution

Researchers at the Institute of HeartMath® (IHM) Research Center in Santa Cruz, California, are exploring the physiological mechanisms by which the heart communicates with the brain. Specifically, they want to understand how communication between the heart (feelings) and the brain (thoughts) influences our perceptions, performance, emotions, behaviors, and health. They hope to learn why we experience the feeling or sensation of love (and other positive emotional states) in the area of the heart and how these feelings affect us physiologically. Also, how do anxiety, stress, and other emotional states affect the autonomic nervous system, the hormonal and immune systems, the heart, and the brain?

Heart rhythms stand out as the best reflection of inner emotional states. Negative emotions lead to increased disorder in the heart's rhythms and in the autonomic nervous system, while positive emotions create increased harmony and coherence in heart rhythms and improve balance in the nervous system.

The HeartMath® researchers have developed techniques that increase coherence in the heart's rhythmic patterns, which then entrains the brain. This results in shifts in perception and in the ability to reduce stress and anxiety, as well as in improving learning and performance. While certain rhythmic breathing exercises will induce coherence, research shows that you can increase these benefits by actively combining positive feelings, such as appreciation, love, and compassion, with your breathing. According to chief researcher Dr. Rollin McCraty, generating a positive emotion makes it easier to sustain coherence for longer periods, even during challenging situations.

Learning to send feelings of love and appreciation throughout your system while breathing as if through your heart adds a dynamic set of benefits to emotional self-management and healing. Many who have tried this exercise describe their experience as an increased ability to "live more from the heart" in alignment with their core values and with greater connection to spirit.

HeartMath® has shown how decision making from the heart can tone down our overactive and often misperceiving brains, with the results being more holistic and, ultimately, more effective. Our modern Western emphasis on the brain instead of the heart may be faulty. Leading with the heart may be the right way to go after all!

For more information, visit www.heartmath.com.

Putting It All Together

How do you incorporate these ideas and practices into your own life? You can begin by being grateful. You know the saying "count your blessings"? Well, do it—literally. We all have a lot to be grateful for. And no matter how bad things might appear, there is always someone who has worse problems. Recall the Hindu expression: "A man who has no shoes is glad he has his feet." In fact, reaching out to those less fortunate will most likely help you at least as much as it helps them. Adult victims of early violence have turned around and helped other survivors, turning their misfortune into a gift to others. The 12-step recovery programs do this well. As individuals share their troubles, those who have "been there" are available to listen and offer support, with healing taking place for all present.

Remember to maintain your sense of humor and perpective. As George Bernard Shaw put it, "Life does not cease to be funny when someone dies, any more than it ceases to be serious when someone laughs."

Positive Programming

- **Resolve an issue you have with someone.** Write a long and thorough letter expressing all your difficult feelings about him or her, going through every emotionally charged incident, holding nothing back. Tell this someone that you won't accept his or her behavior. Don't send the letter. Now, write a letter detailing everything you like about that person, how much you've learned from him or her, going through every incident you can recall where you felt uplifted and supported by that person. Don't send that letter either. This simple exercise will make you clearer and more able to meet with this person to resolve the issue. In fact, when you're done with this exercise, you may have lost the entire emotional charge and can just laugh off whatever it was that was bothering you.
- **Say how you feel.** When someone asks you how you are, tell them how you *really* feel, not just the usual "good, fine, or great." When you have an emotional charge with someone, you can tell them that "When you said or did 'X,' I felt 'Y,' and I would prefer that you do or say 'Z.'" If you're angry about something, beat up a pillow, go kick boxing, scream your head off or whatever you need to do to get it out of your system in the privacy of your own home.
- **Create your own reality.** While in a state of deep relaxation, visualize what you want to happen. This actually draws the experience to you by keeping you focused on your ideal goal.
- **Be heart-centered.** Instead of always "using your head," try thinking, feeling, visualizing, and sharing from your heart. Send positive, loving feelings to yourself and others.

We are fortunate to have many resources that can help in the process of positive thinking. You can work, one on one, with a psychotherapist or take courses specifically designed to help you work through and move beyond self-limiting negative patterns. You also can read books on the subject. There is something for everyone. See the Recommended Reading and Resources for some of our favorites, based on both our experiences and feedback from others.

16

The Power of Touch

We've all heard about the healing powers of human touch. But what we didn't know until recently was that a lack of touch can impair brain development and may even hasten death. Years ago, psychologists observing babies in orphanages noted that, though the infants were well fed and given rudimentary care, many of them simply wasted away and died. They realized that the only missing ingredient was touch. The staff workers at the orphanages were very limited, and no one had time to hold and cuddle these babies. The babies who did manage to survive this lack of physical closeness were left emotionally and physically stunted for life.

The role of touch in infant development was elegantly demonstrated in a classic test with monkeys. Scientists first isolated baby monkeys in cages. Then the babies were offered two surrogate "mothers": one, a wire form with a rubber nipple that delivered milk, and the second, a terry-cloth form that did not feed them. When the little monkeys were frightened, it was the cloth surrogate that they approached and clung to for comfort. So cuddles appear to be as vital as food!

Modern research has revealed important changes in brain chemistry that occur when animals and children are touched. Those deprived of touch develop chronically high levels of the stress hormone, cortisol, and show corresponding problems with development and learning. Researchers have shown that stroking actually reduces cortisol levels and enhances brain development, according to Harvard researcher Mary Carlson.

Of course the vast majority of us know how wonderful it feels to be held in someone's arms. We don't need scientific reports to know that touch nurtures our bodies and souls. By raising our endorphin levels, human touch can lift us into a state of bliss. Any mother calming a frightened child could tell us this.

And it's not just hugs and caresses that can help us here. Massage has been an integral part of healing practices all over the world for centuries. Western medicine has lost the art of touch, though it is gaining an increased recognition these days. In fact, researchers at Miami, Duke, and Harvard Universities and at Miami's Touch Research Institute have conducted numerous controlled studies that show that massage offers remarkable benefits for treating a whole host of conditions. For example, when premature infants were massaged three times a day for ten days, they gained weight 47 percent faster than other infants. Although both groups of babies consumed the same amounts of formula, the massaged babies appeared better able to absorb and utilize it.

At Columbia Presbyterian Hospital, under the leadership of the innovative heart specialist Dr. Mehmet Oz, massage is offered regularly to patients following open heart surgery and heart transplants. The results show that healing time and complications are greatly reduced. In Dr. Oz's inspiring book *Healing from the Heart,* he reports one case where he was able to resuscitate the failing heart of a young patient just out of cardiac surgery. Unresponsive to the usual efforts, the patient rallied when the doctor massaged his feet vigorously for 45 minutes. This upholds a major finding of reflexology, which is that acupressure points related to all parts of the body are clustered thickly on the soles of the feet. Oz was helping the patient's heart along by stimulating the right point on his feet!

Try this simple exercise: Hold your partner's hand in both of yours, and concentrate on what you feel—the warmth, the contours, and the subtle pulsation of blood flow. Let go after a few minutes and ask your partner how his or her hand feels, compared with the other one. Invariably, the touched hand feels more vibrant, alive, and energized, as if it had been massaged. And you accomplished that with no movement at all!

The Magic of Massage

Rachel, a forty-two-year-old writer, recounts the following adventure that illustrates the magic of receiving and connecting through massage:

> I had an amazing massage experience at the Esalen Institute in Big Sur, California. There was a blue sky above, green mountains in the background, and the azure ocean below, stretching as far as the eye could see. I was already feeling pretty good (and who wouldn't, in this place?) when I entered the massage room. In the background was music that almost instantly calmed my mind and nurtured my spirit. The therapist introduced himself, and I knew from the first touch that this was going to be special.
>
> I could feel the energy flow from his hand, and back from my body in response, and so it continued—a positive feedback loop of bliss! My breathing and heart rate slowed down, the tight muscles in my body surrendered, and my mind was silenced, far from its usual preoccupations. Time disappeared, as we did a silent, intimate tango over the next hour. This delicious dance came to a gentle end—too soon, of course. When we said good-bye, he confided to me that, after four years, this was his last massage there. He was leaving that day, and he had really put his heart and soul into this special occasion.

The very special and intimate nature of such massage raises a question regarding possible sexual overtones, especially when a man is giving a massage to a woman (and vice versa). This issue comes up frequently with those who haven't had much experience with massage. The answer is that the experience did have a sensual aspect to it. When asked about it, Rachel responded that, in fact, she had felt alive and in deep contact with her masseur throughout her body. And, beyond that, with the cosmos. But it did not seem personal to her: it was a different level of connection.

Coming back to earth, now let's address the issue of sexuality versus sensuality. Children and animals are uninhibited in experiencing their sensuality. Cats stretch and love to be stroked. And giggling kids will unabashedly tickle one another, until socialized out of this spontaneity. Sensuality is a natural expression of who we are and does not necessarily lead to sex.

In choosing a massage partner, or even in sharing a hug, be aware that the issue of sexuality may arise. The best approach here is to be sure that clear boundaries and intentions are in place before you begin. In our culture, because touch is not as integral a part of life (as it is in much of the rest of the world), we may confuse it with sexuality. During sex may be the only time many people have physical contact. This leaves out the many people who are without partners, without sexual opportunities, or, even, without a desire for sex. But they may well want, and certainly need, to be touched and hugged.

Terry, a radio show host, relates the following experience:

> A couple of years ago, I was visiting my ninety-eight-year-old grandmother. She was still sharp but severely limited by her poor hearing, sight, and mobility. As we talked quietly—as quietly as you can talk to the near-deaf—I gently rubbed her back. She became nearly tearful, as she thanked me and told me how good that felt. I don't recall if she said directly that she didn't get touched enough, but it was clear to me.
>
> The two things that stick with me are, first, the bond created between us in the way her body being touched also touched her heart. I felt that it awoke something from years before, perhaps even from her youth. And, second, I realized that this moment is waiting to happen for millions of seniors, millions of our mothers and fathers.

The healing power of touch knows no age limits. Now, with permission, go touch someone you love, of any age.

Give, Receive, or Keep It All for Yourself

Learning how to massage is like learning to play a musical instrument. Once you master the basic notes and chords, you can then improvise and let the music come from within. Your movements are the technique, the body you massage the instrument, and it's the interaction between the two that makes the music. The communication is intimate, almost sacred, as your two consciousnesses connect. As the one giving a massage, be sensitive and tune in to your partner. And don't assume you have to be an expert. Even professionals will check in repeatedly—not only verbally but also more subtly by watching body language. When in doubt, ask the person for feedback.

When you're receiving a massage, the first moment of physical contact tells you a lot about what's to come. This moment can be almost sacred when the massage therapist is closely attuned to you and your body. This shared meeting with another human being just doesn't happen often enough in our fast and stressful modern world.

Take advantage of this initial contact by tuning in especially closely to what's happening in your own body while picking up information about the person who is touching you. Focus on your breathing and on relaxing. Rapport and receptivity can be enhanced when the giver and the receiver synchronize their rhythms, both through breathing in sync and by playing soothing background music.

As each part of your body is touched, remember to breathe into it, picturing the tension melting away, releasing more and more deeply with each breath. Communicate about what feels good (or not)—"that feels good, but could you do it a little more lightly?" or "a little stronger" or "lower" or "higher . . ." You get the picture. The key here is to really allow yourself to receive—totally and without guilt.

What if you live alone and don't have access to a massage partner or therapist? Self-massage is an excellent option. Massage your own hands and feet, for example. Put on some music, light a candle, use aromatic oils, and you are off and running (or, actually, the opposite). You may be surprised at how relaxing, even blissful, self-massage can be. Another option is to trade massages with a friend or relative.

What if you're short on time? Exchange foot rubs or back rubs. It does not have to be a full body, one-hour session for you to benefit.

Remember, whether you're the giver or receiver, the key is to connect. We all have a huge capacity to give and receive. The secret is the awareness of this potential gift, the willingness to surrender to it, and the belief that we deserve to feel this good!

Necessities for an At-home Massage

You can create your own special "Massage Temple" setting with the follow-ing suggested necessities:

- A quiet, private, comfortable room.
- A massage table, floor mat, appropriately padded table, or simply a bed. Use a bed only with an intimate partner or with someone who understands the appropriate boundaries.
- Massage oil—apricot, almond, or other natural oil product. We recommend that you avoid petroleum-based products, which are unhealthy.
- Music (see the list on pages 271–272).
- Candles or a dim light.
- Incense or essential oils (see Chapter 18).

17

Sexual Chemistry

One of the most pleasurable highs we can experience, in all its many forms and flavors, is sex. Sex can be soft, warm, and cuddly; wild and passionate; or divinely spiritual. Or it can be all of these at once. Let's have a look at the full array of sensuality and sexuality—fantasy, lust, love, tenderness, and passion. While we won't pretend we have all the answers to this great mystery called sex (who does?), we can describe its range, its effects, ways to enjoy and enhance it, and its accompanying brain and body chemistry.

Sex is as complex as we are, shifting with our moods, our ages, the perfume of that amazing-looking young waitress, or the smile of a man who just strolled by. A "certain look" from your lover from across the room might get you more turned on than actual sexual contact. What is this mystery called *sex*?

Sex in all of its variations permeates every aspect of human life. And like animals—lacking an awareness of reproduction and driven solely by pleasure—humans do not mate for procreation only. Dolphins, for example, display a wide range of sensuality and sexuality in their playful interactions and will even include unsuspecting human beings who are innocently swimming near them. Women have reported being pursued relentlessly by male dolphins who rub themselves unashamedly against their skin, and appear to want more.

The Chemistry of Sex: Hormone Heaven

There are many hormones and neurotransmitters that orchestrate the complex sexual dance, in all its shadings. The following are the major players.

DHEA is an antiaging, energizing, antistress adrenal hormone that can also convert to both estrogen and testosterone. Not only does it stimulate the sexual response, it even stimulates the production of pheromones. As we will reveal in Chapter 18, these are special chemicals secreted by the skin in order to attract the opposite sex via the sense of smell. We can enhance the effect of our pheromones by wearing them in combination with certain essential oils, such as ylang-ylang, vanilla, and musk.

Meanwhile, the pituitary gland, located in the brain, secretes three hormones, each with its own role in this drama: oxytocin, prolactin, and vasopressin. The "bonding hormone," oxytocin, makes couples want to touch and cuddle and contributes to monogamy. In women, it leads to the contractions of orgasm, and in men it speeds ejaculation and promotes a postorgasmic relaxation response, followed all too rapidly by sleep. Prolactin, which is also released during nursing, increases during orgasm, then dips. Vasopressin, especially in men, helps them to maintain mental focus, pick up on sexual clues, and avoid extreme behaviors, such as getting distracted by other women in mid-flirtation. (That often happens anyway, vasopressin notwithstanding.)

The feel-good neurotransmitter phenethylamine (PEA), also found in chocolate, is the "love chemical." It helps to create a feeling of excitement and turn-on. In men, visual cues will set it off, and lust is born. Then along comes the motivator, dopamine, urging a man to ask for a woman's phone number. His fantasies about her raise his level of testosterone, the male sex hormone. This hormone cocktail shunts his rational mind due south. (Testosterone also drives female libido.) As women approach menopause, a decrease in levels of testosterone is a major factor behind decreased sexual desire. Then there are the endorphins, which kick in during and especially just after orgasm, and ecstatic feelings prevail.

We have just caught a glimpse of the complex chemical orchestra that makes all kinds of music, changing volume, beat, and harmony as the various hormonal instruments move into and out of prominence. How can we best preserve and enjoy this symphony and use it for our elevation?

Good sex is high up on the list of natural highs, both as a relaxant and as a means to connection. The more you are in the moment, tuning in to all your senses and sensations, the better the experience. This harkens back to ancient cultures, where sacred sexuality was honored, as opposed to Western society's artificial schism between sex and spirit. The split has led to guilt for having these normal inclinations and even to repression of desire.

In practicing sacred sexuality, we have an opportunity to reconnect with ourselves and our partners in a very deep and powerful way. This not only renews and reenergizes us but also brings us closer to the essence of who we are. This practice can enhance creativity, love, knowledge, empowerment, passion, and a celebration of life. To quote Margo Anand, author of *The Art of Sexual Ecstasy,* "Ecstasy transcends sex. Every moment is pregnant with ecstasy."

Don't forget to play. Sex is one area where we can also be playful, silly, creative, and spontaneous. Despite all the serious aspects that we just discussed, don't forget to just have a good time—on your own or with a partner.

Sex can't exactly be orchestrated. As in learning to dance, the right moves will become second nature, and you will discover all kinds of creative things to do. There are also many tapes and books that give you a series of exercises that build on one another to help expand your range of sexual feelings and repertoire of activities. Here are some guidelines for creating a conducive atmosphere. Your own preferences will, of course, work the best.

1. Sex is not limited to physical sexual contact or to the bedroom. Set the stage far in advance.
2. Leave a love note for your partner, inviting him or her to a mysterious evening encounter. Send him or her flowers during the day. Leave a provocative message on your partner's answering machine.

3. Have a candle-lit dinner and play romantic music in the back-ground. Serve finger food that you can feed lovingly to each other. (Don't stop to do the dishes!)

4. Take a bubble bath scented with essential oil aphrodisiacs, such as vanilla, musk, or ylang-ylang. Use a candle to light the bathroom.

5. Maintain eye contact as much as you can (without tripping on the stairs) and feel the charge building up between you.

6. By the time you reach the bedroom, you will have been engaged in sex for hours! Try a slow massage—hands, feet, back, and neck. You might want to play more rhythmic music at this point.

7. You get the picture. Sex is much more meaningful and enjoy-able if you can move beyond the physical act.

18

Aromatherapy

Fragrance captures our attention: the aroma of freshly baked bread, the sweet smell of a rose, or the scent of a cup of warm peppermint tea. We are drawn to certain smells that remind us of happy times—the cinnamon and cloves of hot apple cider at Christmas, the scent of pinewoods, or the salty tang of the sea. A special key to conjuring up images of the past, smell evokes emotions and memories like no other sense can.

The Knowing Nose

How does smell affect us so deeply and immediately? This most basic of all senses is vital for survival in the animal world—whether searching for food, sniffing for danger, or seeking a mate. Smells are carried directly by the olfactory nerves to the limbic system, a primitive part of the brain that acts as a kind of emotional switchboard. The limbic system evaluates sensory stimuli, registering pleasure or pain, safety or danger, and then directs our corresponding emotional responses, such as anger, fear, repulsion, or attraction. This response then connects to the part of the brain that influences memory, learning, basic emotions, hormonal balances, and even our basic survival mechanisms, such as the "fight or flight" response.

Because smell has the longest recall of all the senses, a particular scent can unlock and help us retrieve specific memories, some many years old, that we associate with that odor. Scents can be a direct pathway to memory and emotion. Fragrances can relieve pain, call up deep-seated memories, and generally affect personality and behavior.

Using oil fragrances may turn out to be one of the fastest ways to achieve psychological results, too. "Smells act directly on the brain, like a drug," says Dr. Alan Hirsch, a neurologist, psychiatrist, and director of the Smell and Taste Treatment and Research Center in Chicago.

Essential Oils and Aromatherapy

The term *aromatherapy* was first coined in the early part of the twentieth century by the French chemist René-Maurice Gattefossé to describe the medicinal use of essential oils. These oils are the vital essence or "soul" of the plant, containing their concentrated therapeutic and nutritional compounds, including phytohormones. Just as in humans, these are chemical messengers that act throughout the plant in response to environmental conditions, including stress. These plant hormones can affect us, too, when we inhale their fragrance, apply them topically, or ingest them. In fact, many traditional herbal remedies had multiple purposes—a single potion often served as a perfume, topical salve, and oral medicine.

Scientific evidence supporting aromatherapy is just beginning to surface. In a 1992 issue of the *British Journal of Occupational Therapy*, aromatherapy is described as a treatment to "promote health and well-being" through massage, inhalation, baths, and the application of compresses, creams, and lotions. This suggests that fragrance can reduce stress and depression, sedate or invigorate, stimulate sensory awareness, and provide pain relief. Researchers have found that fragrance can even improve human interaction and communication: pleasant smells can put people in better moods and make them more willing to negotiate, cooperate, and compromise than they would be in a scent-free room.

Oil on Troubled Waters

Different scents produce specific emotional states, communicated through the various neurotransmitters. Marjoram oil, for example, is a sedating oil that stimulates the secretion of the calming transmitter serotonin. Dr. J. J. King, a psychiatrist at the Smallwood Day Hospital in Redditch, Worcestershire, has successfully treated anxiety with pleasant, natural scents that are known relaxants, including lavender, rose, bergamot, cypress, and balsam fir. He also combines these with relaxation techniques, such as deep breathing, positive visualization, soothing music, and heat treatments. Once patients learn to associate a particular fragrance with deep relaxation, they relax whenever they are given a sniff. In addition to the intrinsic qualities of the oils themselves, then, he has added a "conditioned response," wherein the body and mind are trained to associate the smell with the relaxed state.

One way to measure this response is to monitor certain brain waves with an electroencephalograph, or EEG. "We know from brain-wave frequency studies that smelling lavender increases alpha waves in the back of the head, which are associated with relaxation," says Dr. Hirsch. The scents that have proved to have the greatest sedative effect have been (in order of effectiveness): lavender, bergamot, marjoram, sandalwood, lemon, and chamomile.

According to research by Dr. Susan Schiffman, professor of medical psychology at Duke University in North Carolina, sedative drugs like Valium and Librium affect a newly discovered group of smell receptors in the brain. She reasons that if smell receptors help to sedate us, the fragrance itself should perform similarly. To test her theory, she sprayed spicy scents into New York City subway cars to see if the scents relaxed the passengers enough to improve their dispositions. After comparing the number of pushes, shoves, and nasty comments in scented cars to those in unscented cars, she found that certain fragrances appeared to cut aggressive acts almost in half. Sounds like an excellent idea!

Refreshing Mood Boosters

Sixteenth- and seventeenth-century herbalists in Europe used clary sage and lemon balm to counter mental fatigue and depression, and they are still used for this purpose today. These simple drug-free antidepressants may eventually be accepted by medical doctors as well. According to recent research by biochemist George Dodd and psychologist Steve van Toller, at the Warwick Olfaction Research Group in England, the effect of fragrance on the brain is similar to that of some antidepressant drugs, implying that certain scents actually alter brain chemistry.

Aromatic Uppers

Long-distance truck drivers and others whose jobs depend on their staying alert can now sniff specific formulas that help them to do so. Train conductors in Japan and Russia use an "odorphone" developed by Russian professor of biology and odorology V. Krasnov. The little machine spews out hot whiffs of pine, cedar, rose, or even seaweed or mushroom, as required. Air New Zealand and Virgin Atlantic airlines have even developed kits available to passengers at London's Heathrow Airport, containing floral-scented bath oils to reduce jet lag.

Some of the first investigation into fragrant stimulants was done in the 1920s by Italian psychiatrists Giovanni Gatti and Renato Cayola. They found that the scents of clove, ylang-ylang, cinnamon, lemon, cardamom, fennel, and angelica were stimulating. American studies through International Flavors and Fragrances (IFF) also found peppermint and eucalyptus to be stimulating. Modern-day research at Toho University School of Medicine in Tokyo showed that these fragrances and numerous others—basil, jasmine, black pepper, and, to a lesser degree, rose, patchouli, lemon grass, and sage—also acted as stimulants. They tend to increases beta waves in the front of the brain associated with a more alert state. Consider sniffing these when studying for exams!

These healthy stimulants do not trigger the stress response but instead actually counter the typical adrenal response caused by caffeine, stress, and other common stimulative triggers. They also relieve drowsiness, irritability, and headaches. Dr. S. Torii has found that, by arousing the autonomic nervous system, which controls breathing and blood pressure, stimulating fragrances help to maintain attention, which generally lags after 30 minutes of sustained concentration.

To test the effects of such fragrances on alertness, University of Cincinnati researchers W. Dember and J. Warm gave people a stressful 40-minute task based on identifying patterns on a computer. Those working in rooms scented with peppermint had many more correct answers than those working in unscented rooms. In addition, their performance levels didn't decline as rapidly. In a study conducted by researchers at Rensselaer Polytechnic Institute in Troy, New York, clerical workers set specific goals for themselves and were more efficient when their offices were specifically scented. The fragrance worked even when those taking the test did not think that the scent was influencing them.

Scent and Sex

Aphrodisiac scents such as jasmine and ylang-ylang stimulate the pituitary gland to secrete endorphins, which relay feelings of relaxation, bliss, and expanded consciousness to our brains.

Some fragrances—including ylang-ylang, rose, patchouli, sandalwood, jasmine, vanilla, and musk—are both relaxing and stimulating. Although it might seem as if these effects would cancel each other out, they actually combine to produce a very enjoyable mood. Since stress and tension are strong deterrents to passion, the state of being completely relaxed yet stimulated offers the perfect combination for an aphrodisiac. Other aphrodisiacs include the stimulants cinnamon and coriander—used for this purpose in *The Arabian Nights*.

The association of scent and sex comes as no surprise. All animals, humans included, utilize the sex-scent "pheromone" molecules to attract or find a potential mate. Produced in specialized apocrine or sweat glands, they are picked up by the tiny vomeronasal organ in the nose. The signal is then transmitted to the limbic system, creating a sexual response. Researchers have exposed people in public places and offices to pheromone extracts. The result was a noticeable increase in friendly behavior. In one experiment, a pair of identical female twins was sent to a singles bar, with only one wearing a pheromone extract. Video cameras capturing the action showed that the scented twin had far more men make overtures while, by comparison, her equally attractive sister was practically a wallflower. And, as in nature, these men had no idea what had hit them.

Transcendent Scents

Life energy—variously known as *chi* in China, *prana* in India, *bioplasma* in Russia, or *vital force* in the parlance of homeopathy—is the metaphysical aspect of the body. Essential oils promote strengthening of this invisible energy field, the aura, in which we exist, and through which we all connect. When combined with the healing touch of massage, essential oils will literally expand the aura, as seen on Kirlian photographs, a method of measuring electrical energy by its image on film. Mystics and spiritual teachers have always known this, and many religious traditions have included the use of essential oils in their rituals. A great source of information on the esoteric aspects of essential oils is Dr. Bruce Berkowsky, who has written several books and gives seminars through the Institute of Natural Health Science. For more information, visit www.naturalhealthscience.com.

Essential Oils: The Essentials

Essential oils are ideal for skin care, massage, and mental and emotional rejuvenation. But some people, especially those allergic to perfumes, may be sensitive to certain essences. You can safely "patch test" essential oils by placing a few drops on the back of your hand. If you develop any redness, itching, or burning, discontinue use.

It's vital to buy good-quality natural essential oils. True essential oils emit full, complex fragrances that are nearly impossible to duplicate in the laboratory. No synthetic copy, regardless of its derivation, can match the precise blend of chemicals found in an essential oil. Even slight changes will unbalance the fragrance and, by upsetting delicate synergies, eliminate or reduce their therapeutic value. The only way to be sure of the quality of a fragrance is to purchase it from a reputable supplier.

You need to blend pure essential oils with "carrier" oils—refined, expeller-pressed vegetable oils, such as almond oil. Add 5 ml (0.2 fl oz) of essential oil to 115 ml (4 fl oz) of carrier oil to produce aromatic oil for massage or perfume. For bath oils, it is better to use half as much carrier oil; blend 5 ml (0.2 fl oz) of essential oil with 60 ml (2 fl oz) of carrier oil. Or, as you will see below, simply add the essential oil to your bathwater.

Here are some good ways to use essential oils:

Massage: To induce relaxation, use lavender, orange, marjoram, or chamomile. To ease muscular pain, use chamomile or lavender. Select the carrier oil according to your skin type: for oily skin use apricot, walnut, or soy; for dry skin, use olive, almond, or cocoa butter; and for normal skin, use corn, sesame, sunflower, or canola.

Bath: Add 6–8 drops of a soothing essence, such as chamomile, rose, orange, lavender, sandalwood, or ylang-ylang, to a hot bath to waft away your troubles.

Room scenting: You can enjoy the psychological benefits of essential oils while refreshing and purifying indoor air by diffusing essences in your room or home with aroma lamps or electric diffusers. Aroma lamps warm essential oils in water over a candle, evaporating their scent into the air. Diffusers emit atomized essential oil and small amounts of deodorizing ozone.

Perfume: Before synthetics, perfumes were made by blending essential oils with vegetable oils and animal scents, such as musk. Make your own perfume by adding a few drops of essence to carrier oil. For attracting the opposite sex, use a pheromone-spiked formula (but be prepared for the consequences!).

You can make aromatherapy blends yourself. The chart below describes some of our favorite blends.

Aromatherapy Blends

Depending on your needs, use one of the following formulas in your bath, for scenting your room or home, as a perfume, or for massage.

RELAXANT FRAGRANCE
4 fl oz sweet almond oil
10 drops each lavender and lemon essential oils
2 drops each marjoram and sandalwood essential oils

MOOD-BOOSTER FRAGRANCE
4 fl oz sweet almond oil
10 drops each bergamot and petitgrain essential oils
3 drops rose geranium essential oil
1 drop neroli essential oil (expensive, so it's optional)

STIMULANT FOR FATIGUE
4 fl oz sweet almond oil
15 drops lemon essential oil
4 drops eucalyptus essential oil
1 drop each cinnamon, peppermint, clove, patchouli, benzoin, and/or sage essential oils (as available)

MEMORY STIMULANT
4 fl oz sweet almond oil
10 drops each lavender and lemon essential oils
5 drops rosemary essential oil
1 drop cinnamon essential oil

APHRODISIAC
4 fl oz sweet almond oil
10 drops each lavender and sandalwood essential oils
2 drops each ylang-ylang and vanilla essential oils
1 drop each cinnamon and jasmine essential oils

(continued)

(Lavender is not an aphrodisiac but is added to make the fragrance more mellow. It can be a relaxing and emotionally uplifting scent. Also, if you love the fragrance of patchouli, you can use it in place of ylang-ylang.)

CONNECT FORMULA

10 drops lavender essential oil

2 drops each mandarin orange, geranium bourbon, ylang-ylang, and patchouli essential oils

19

The Music of the Emotions

Music has charms to soothe a savage breast.
WILLIAM CONGREVE (1670–1729)

Half an hour of music produces the same effect as ten milligrams of Valium.
RAYMOND BAHR, DIRECTOR OF CORONARY CARE,
ST. AGNES HOSPITAL, BALTIMORE, MARYLAND

You know how a special song can transport you back in time, to take you to a very specific experience, one that you can actually feel in your body? Think of a hit song from your teenage years, a period in your life when you were beginning to experience so many new aspects of the world. Does the song get your emotions—or your hormones—flowing again? Can you feel your heart breaking all over again when you hear a song that was playing when you split up with your first love? Or, on a more up note, does your heart open wide when you hear the strains of "Ode to Joy" from Beethoven's Ninth Symphony?

Music is a powerful key to our bodies and psyches. Although its role in the West is largely entertainment, for thousands of years people throughout the world have used music to heal the body, mind, and spirit. The field of "sound healing" has begun to emerge once again into public awareness. Recent studies have shown that music can reduce stress, enhance immune system function, slow down (and even balance) brain-wave activity, reduce muscle tension, increase endorphin levels, and evoke feelings of love and inner peace. Pretty good for something as available as your nearest CD player or radio!

267

We've Got Rhythm

Although there are many paths to healing, the common denominator in most techniques is that the body is best able to heal itself when in a state of deep relaxation. And by relaxation we don't mean simply "doing nothing" or "vegging out" in front of the TV. People may *think* they are achieving meaningful relaxation, but they are often mistaken. Specific relaxation techniques are usually necessary.

One of the simplest and most effective ways to evoke the *relaxation response,* a term coined by Dr. Herbert Benson in his landmark book of the same name, is through the use of music. The most powerful effect of music is our physical response to "the beat." The phenomenon known as *rhythm entrainment* describes how an external rhythmic stimulus, such as a ticking clock, drum, or pulse in a musical composition, involuntarily causes your heartbeat to match its speed.

Innovative New Age composer Steven Halpern has been a leader and researcher in the field of sound and healing since 1970. He writes:

> At age 22, I was already a classic Type A individual. Given my background as an ex–New Yorker, it was not surprising that my requirement was "I want my relaxation—and I want it now!" I needed a solution—something legal, non-addictive and effective, available at my convenience and virtually instantaneous. (Does this sound familiar?) The solution was to combine my training in music and psychology with insights ranging from ancient shamanic sound traditions to modern bio-physics and vibrational medicine.

We now have an extensive body of research that has measured and validated the psychological and physiological benefits of music on human development and behavior. For example, the electromagnetic field surrounding our head literally entrains and attunes to the basic electromagnetic field of the earth itself in a state of deep relaxation or meditation! The earth's harmonic resonance has been measured at approximately 8 cycles per second, or 8 hertz (Hz). The frequency range of the electrical activity of the brain that we access in states of deep relaxation is also centered around 8 Hz.

This is why we feel so rejuvenated when surrounded by nature—in a forest, in the mountains, or near the ocean.

Music has the power to restore our connection with our essence and with the cosmos. According to Halpern, who was among the first to use sound and music to induce relaxation and shift brain waves into alpha and theta states, "Being in harmony with oneself and the Universe may be more than a poetic concept." It is in the stillness that we align and attune to the deeper spiritual dimensions of life. It is in the stillness that true healing occurs. There is no need to "do" anything; all you need is to "be" with the music. For more information, visit www.innerpeacemusic.com.

The Chemistry of Sound

At the Addiction Research Center in Stanford, California, people listened to various kinds of music, including marching bands, spiritual anthems, and movie soundtracks. About half the listeners reported feelings of euphoria, leading the researchers to suspect that the joy of music is linked to the release of endorphins. To test this theory, investigators injected listeners with naloxone, which blocks opiate (endorphin) receptors. Sure enough, the listeners experienced far less pleasure. This suggests that certain types of music can actually boost endorphins.

There is also research on the effects of music on stress levels. Clinical psychologist and music therapist Mark Rider tested cortisol levels of twelve shift-working nurses under high stress. As you may recall, cortisol is secreted by the adrenal glands during the "fight or flight" stress response. He also took body temperatures to assess the degree to which the nurses' bodies retained proper circadian (day/night) rhythms—an indicator of body-mind homeostasis or inner balance. When the nurses listened to tapes of soothing music and practiced relaxation and guided imagery, their rhythms were appropriately balanced, and their levels of stress hormones were reduced. On days when the nurses did not listen to the tapes, their rhythms were out of balance, and their stress hormones were significantly higher.

This is reflected in the words of Dr. Mitchell Gaynor in *Sounds of Healing*:

> *I am convinced that each of us has our own perfect, inborn biofeedback monitor that tells us which sound waves have the most salutary influence on our cardiovascular, immune and nervous systems, not to mention our emotional and spiritual selves.*

Composer and author Joshua Leeds describes how various combinations of sounds can create specific effects in the brain, including speeding it up or slowing it down. His series of CDs allows you to change your own rhythm just by turning them on and tuning in. For more information, visit www.sound-remedies.com.

Ecstasy through Music

Relaxation is not the only pleasurable state that music can induce. When we can't stop pulsating along with the insistent beat of a samba, or keep from leaping up from our seats at a rock concert, we are responding to the power of music to literally move us. From chanting dervishes, who whirl their way into ecstatic dance, to young clubbers, we are all doing what comes naturally. Feeling down? Put on an upbeat CD, and let the beat take over. Here is a quote from Joel S., a forty-five-year-old successful "business activist" and sometime drummer:

> *I find drumming a deep cleansing, a harmonization and alignment of my cellular structure with the rhythm and groove. If people are dancing, I need to consciously relax, breathe, and allow the energy to go through me—or I will explode. Then, I end up smiling uncontrollably—both while I'm drumming and for some time afterward. I'm high!*

You can consciously alter your mental state by using music—as a natural stimulant, a relaxant, a mood booster, and a connector—both at home and at work. Relaxation and work are not contradictory concepts. Many people spend 45 percent or more of their waking state in their offices, and the demand for efficiency and effectiveness continues to grow. Using the right musical background can actually promote your productivity and creativity, while simultaneously maintaining your energy and uplifting your sense of overall well-being.

The chart below provides some musical selections that will help you to relax or stimulate or uplift your mood and sense of connection. We are sure you have your own, too (R = relaxing, S = stimulating, U = uplifting).

Type	Artist(s)	Title	Source/More Information
MAINLY INSTRUMENTAL			
R/U	Siddha Yoga	*Remembrance*	www.siddhayoga.org
R/U	Peter Gabriel	*Passion*	Uni/Geffen
U	Mark Knopfler	*Screenplaying*	Warner Brothers
R	Paul Horn	*Inside Taj Mahal*	Kuckuck Records
R/U	Robert Gass	*Pilgrimage*	Spring Hill Music
R/U	Steven Halpern	*Gifts of the Angels* (and others)	www.innerpeacemusic.com
R/U	Gabrielle Roth	*Totem & Refuge*	www.ravenrecording.com
CHORAL			
R/U	Salva Regina	*Gregorian Chant*	Phillips International
U	Voices of Ascension	*Beyond Chant*	Delos delosmus.com
U	Robert Gass	*Songs of Healing*	Spring Hill Music
WORLD MUSIC			
U	Henri Dikongue	*C'est la vie* (African)	www.worldmusic.com/tinder
U	Boy Ge Mendes	*Lagoa* (Brazilian)	www.worldmusic.com/tinder
U	Sting	Fields of Gold	A & M Records
S/U	Govi	*Andalusian Nights* (Flamenco)	Higher Octave (1999)

(continued)

WORLD MUSIC (*continued*)			
S/U	Buena Vista Social Club	*Buena Vista Social Club* (Cuban)	Discos Corazón

ELECTRONIC/KEYBOARD/VOCALS			
S/U	Enigma	*Love, Sensuality, Devotion*	Virgin
R/U	Andreas Vollenveider	*Down to the Moon*	Sony
S/R	Compilation	*Euphoria/Chilled*	www.telstar.co.uk
S/U	Lost at Last	*Ocean of Mercy/ Lost at Last*	www.lostatlast.com
S/U	Lisa Gerrard	*Duality*	4AD
S/U	Loreena McKennitt	*The Book of Secrets*	Warner Brothers
S	Soundtrack	*Better Living through Circuitry*	www.moonshine.com
R	Cafe del Mar	*5 & 7*	Mercury Records
S/R	Compilation	*The Chillout Album* (1 & 2)	www.telstar.co.uk

CLASSICAL			
R/U	Compilation	*Shadows and Light*	Deutsche Grammophon (1995)
R/U	Albinoni/ Pachelbel	Adagios	Warner Classics (1996)
R/U	Dvorak	*New World Symphony*	Essential Classics
R/U	Brahms	Symphony No. 4	Classical Navigator
S	J. S. Bach	*Brandenburg Concertos*	Pearl
S	Handel	*Water Music Suite, Music for the Royal Fireworks*	Columbia
S/U	Beethoven	Fourth, Fifth, and Ninth Symphonies	EMI
S/U	Vivaldi	*Four Seasons* ("Spring" and "Summer")	Eloquence

20

Light and Color

A Stimulating Light

Ever wonder why a vacation in the sun leaves you feeling so high? It might all boil down to the positive effects of natural sunlight. Many people suffer from light deficiency. Some are more susceptible than others and consequently are more prone to low moods, especially in the winter. There is now plenty of evidence that by increasing light exposure you can boost your mental performance as well as your mood.

One of the pioneers of light therapy was the late Francis Lefebure, who developed a technique known as *phosphenism*. The afterimages that are seen when you close your eyes after looking at a light source are called *phosphenes*. He studied this phenomenon and was able to demonstrate that various exercises that involved closing your eyes and focusing on these afterimages could stimulate learning, mood, motivation, and creativity. Unfortunately, despite impressive results, his work has not been followed up. We include one very simple phosphenic exercise at the end of this chapter that can be very helpful for those prone to low moods, especially during the winter.

Light also stimulates skin cells to produce a powerful immune-boosting substance called *interleukin-1 (IL-1)*. Since it is stimulated by natural daylight, you have good reason to spend some time every day outdoors exposing yourself, so to speak.

What makes natural sunlight different from indoor lighting? Natural sunlight contains the full spectrum of wavelengths that we perceive as "white" light. Pass sunlight through a prism (or rain droplets) and it separates into a rainbow, revealing the wide range of wavelengths provided by natural light. Indoor lighting, by contrast, uses lightbulbs that provide a limited range of wavelengths. Regular incandescent bulbs tend to provide illumination with a yellow cast. Fluorescent lighting comes a bit closer to sunlight, but the tendency for fluorescent lights to flicker makes them less desirable. The best indoor lighting, called "full-spectrum" lighting, aims to mimic all of the wavelengths of natural light and, likewise, to reproduce all of its benefits. If you work indoors with little exposure to natural light, it's worth investing in full-spectrum lighting. (See Resources for a list of suppliers.)

A Healthy Color

Colors influence your mood. Research in schools investigating the effects of changing the colors in classrooms has shown that yellow, orange, and red increase IQ and stimulate learning, while black and brown have the opposite effect, and green is neutral. Blue has been shown to calm down hyperactive children. The effects of exposing yourself to different hues of light is likely to be even more powerful. Color is used in a variety of ways for healing. Although color therapists stress that everyone responds to colors differently, the following colors will tend to have the following effects:

Violet—Connects. Peaceful. Meditative. Helps balance the mind.
Magenta—Connects. Energizes. Empowers.
Blue—Relaxes. Calms body and mind. Antidote to stress.
Turquoise—Relaxes. Soothing. Refreshing. Eases anxiety.
Orange—Stimulates. Enhances cheerful mood. Relaxes.
Red—Stimulates. Invigorates. Activates. Relieves exhaustion.
White—Stimulates. Boosts mood. Enhances mind and connection.

You can put this information to good use by having "soft" lights for your evening lighting that emit turquoise, blue, magenta, or violet color ranges. Candlelight, which is of a much lower intensity, is also much more calming than strong daylight. For your "day" lighting, make sure you have plenty of light, either as natural daylight or full-spectrum lightbulbs.

Light Exercise

This exercise is particularly effective for those prone to depression, especially during the winter when there is less natural daylight.

1. Sit down in a quiet place, on the floor or on a chair. It is best to choose a place that you can completely darken. If not, you will need a blindfold.
2. Place an angle-poise lamp, containing a 60-watt opaque (not clear) bulb, preferably with no writing on it, three feet away and directly in line with your line of vision.
3. Make sure you can turn the light on and off without moving the position of your head.
4. Turn the light on and look directly at the bulb for 1 minute, no longer.
5. After 1 minute, turn the light off, close your eyes (put on your blindfold if the room is not completely dark), and focus on the after-image, the phosphene, without moving your head, until it completely vanishes. This usually takes 3 to 4 minutes.

There are also special full-spectrum lighting systems called SAD (seasonal affective disorder) lights. Their use in winter is a great way to chase the winter blahs (unless you happen to live in Florida). Check Resources for a list of suppliers.

21

Deep Sleep

A good snooze is one of the cheapest, safest, most available, and most natural highs going. According to experts, if you want to be fully alert, cheerful, mentally sharp, creative, and energetic all day, you need to spend about eight hours a night, or one-third of your life, asleep.

"People have no idea how important sleep is to their lives," says Thomas Roth, Health and Scientific Advisor of the National Sleep Foundation. "Good health demands good sleep. Conversely, lack of sleep and sleep problems have serious, often life-threatening consequences."

Why do we need so much sleep? Our bodies are governed by the circadian cycle in response to the cyclic rhythms of the sun moving through night and day, and shifting with the changing seasons. The circadian cycle, in turn, acts as an internal clock to coordinate our inner rhythms in areas such as hormone production, mood, body temperature, and energy level. To maintain the dynamic balance of all these systems, we need to spend sufficient time sleeping. And we are not alone in this—nearly all animals and even some plants sleep on a regular basis, repairing and rejuvenating themselves during this dormant period.

Just like the overused stress response, the genetic blueprint for sleep has not evolved quickly enough to keep pace with our emerging twenty-four-hour-a-day lives. Before the electric lightbulb extended our days, most people slept an average of ten hours a night. In the 1950s and 1960s, this dropped to about eight hours. It now hovers around seven and continues to fall. More than one in three people boast of sleeping six hours or less.

Loss of sleep has its price. Even minimal sleep loss makes us less alert and attentive, and more moody and irritable. As our concentration and judgment wane and our ability to perform even simple tasks declines, our true productivity shrinks. At the same time, accident rates increase, as do health problems, especially in our gastrointestinal, cardiovascular, hormonal, and immune systems. Our relationships suffer, too.

Pointing to our escalating pace of life, work pressures, and aging, many medical specialists now believe sleep disorders to be a major health problem. Disturbed sleep reflects and affects everything else that goes on in our bodies and minds. The ancient Chinese and other traditional medical systems knew to account for these cycles in both diagnosis and treatment.

Insomnia and the Stress Response

Researchers have found that insomniacs with the highest degree of sleep disturbance secrete the highest amounts of cortisol—particularly in the evening and night-time hours—which prevents them from sleeping. They concluded that chronic insomnia is a disorder of hyperarousal present throughout the twenty-four-hour sleep/wake cycle. As we discussed previously, the increased production of stress hormones is likely to lead to depression and contributes to the development of high blood pressure, obesity, and osteoporosis. Thus, activities that reduce these dangerous stress-hormone levels will promote both sleep and improved health.

Activities that can help control damaging stress-hormone levels include exercise, meditation, and emotional-release techniques, such as Gary Craig's self-administered Emotional Freedom Technique (EFT), which is explained on the Web site www.emofree.com; or Francine Shapiro's Eye Movement Desensitization and Reprocessing (EMDR), which is explained on the Web site www.emdr.org.

REM Sleep: A Chance to Dream

Sleep is a complex and dynamic process with its own rhythms. Sleep labs monitor these patterns through the use of an electroencephalograph, or EEG. Electrodes are attached to specific locations on a subject's scalp, and physiological changes are recorded on graph paper in a series of jagged lines. Specialists can tell which stage of sleep someone is in and, by reviewing a full night's recording, whether or not the individual has a normal sleep cycle.

After about half an hour, sleep becomes physically restorative as cells start to repair and rejuvenate. In an hour or so, sleep shifts into the highly active stage called REM sleep, characterized by accelerated dreaming and rapid eye movements (REM). Though some may dream in all stages of sleep, dreams occur most frequently in REM sleep and are usually more vivid and emotional than during other stages. For most adults, REM sleep occurs every 90 minutes throughout the night. As the night progresses, REM periods become longer, lasting up to 30 to 45 minutes and dominating the sleep cycle. This pattern, with the longer REM period coming at the end of the sleep cycle, offers one of the clearest arguments for getting at least seven to eight hours of sleep per night.

During REM sleep, the brain replenishes its supply of neurotransmitters, such as noradrenaline and serotonin, that are crucial for new learning and retention as well as for mood. REM sleep also allows the subconscious mind to analyze the day's events and process feelings, an essential activity for mental health. In fact, REM sleep is rather like running a cleanup program on your computer. During the day, we generate a lot of open and disconnected circuits, and probably end up with plenty of fragmented and corrupted files. Unless we run our nightly cleanup, the next day our human computer is likely to run slower and less efficiently, to say nothing of the occasional system errors and total crashes. Thus, adequate REM sleep is vital for memory storage, retention, mental organization, new learning, and emotional balance.

Recent experiments led by Dr. Robert Stickgold at Harvard Medical School demonstrated how important sleep is to our ability to retain new learning. The experiments point to a new theory of memory formation that involves interaction between two stages of sleep—one that occurs at the beginning of the night and one that occurs early in the morning. When people learn a new skill, their performance does not improve until after they have had more than six, and preferably eight, hours of sleep.

Without adequate sleep, the brain may not be able to properly encode skills and even new factual information into its memory circuits. In fact, a person's intelligence may be less important than a good night's sleep for forming many kinds of memories. Cramming all night before final exams, then, may get you through the next day (on an adrenaline high), but you are likely to forget most of what you learned.

A recent study found that increased REM sleep time is also an excellent mood enhancer. Just think of all the prescriptions written for neurotransmitter-enhancing antidepressants, or sleeping pills, when the underlying problem is actually sleep deprivation. In fact, many of these drugs may actually suppress REM sleep and reduce the supply of available neurotransmitters, thereby aggravating low moods.

You can see now why REM deficiency, sleep deprivation, and fatigue often develop into a self-perpetuating cycle: Decreased sleep reduces REM; reduced REM prevents rejuvenation; unrejuvenated, we are more susceptible to stress; feeling stressed decreases sleep. Add sleeping pills to the mix, and you just increase the problem. These drugs basically knock us unconscious, then rob us of our precious restorative REM sleep.

Natural Sleep Aids: And So to Bed

Having created a social epidemic of sleep deprivation, we need now to turn away from these REM-suppressing drugs. Fortunately, we have a choice of herbs that have been shown not only to promote calm and well-being but also to act as an effective natural treatment for insomnia. These herbs are able to bring on deep restful sleep without interfering with our natural cycles. They include kava, valerian, hops, passionflower, and reishi mushroom. These herbs were discussed in Chapters 4 and 5.

Sleep disorders are sometimes linked with lowered brain levels of the neurotransmitter serotonin and its metabolite melatonin. The herb St. John's wort has both serotonin- and melatonin-enhancing effects, making it an excellent sleep regulator. Many of our patients notice that their sleep improves markedly after just a few weeks on St. John's wort. Another choice is 5-hydroxytryptophan (5-HTP), which enhances sleep by increasing serotonin levels. Try 50 mg of 5-HTP one hour before bedtime. If that doesn't work, increase to 100 mg or a maximum of 200 mg daily.

The hormone melatonin is another important aid to sleep, which is instrumental in establishing our daily rhythms. As we age, our melatonin levels decrease, with the steepest decline occurring after age fifty. Melatonin supplements may play a role in restoring internal sleeping and waking rhythms by working on the underlying physiological causes of sleep disorder. In one study using melatonin, men and women between the ages of sixty-eight and eighty fell asleep in half their usual time. They also reported that their sleep was more refreshing.

If you want to try melatonin, begin with 1 mg the first night, and if it works, continue with that dose. If not, try increasing the dose by 1 mg each night, but only up to a maximum of 5 mg daily. If you wake up feeling groggy or if you have dreams that are overly stimulating, cut back. Your internal clock should be reset after about two weeks, at which point you can discontinue the melatonin. While its popularity has increased due to its possible antiaging effects, melatonin is still a hormone and needs to be used with appropriate caution, as noted.

Taking supplements and sleep aids is only one way of bringing on that moment when, after a long day of myriad responsibilities and stresses, you collapse into bed, crawl under the cozy covers, and finally sink into sleep. A good night's sleep is an art that you can learn. The following suggestions have been proven to promote healthy sleep:

- Develop a routine. Try to wake up and go to bed at the same time each day. Irregular bedtimes and waking times are not conducive to a good night's sleep.
- Avoid stimulants in the evening and, ideally, throughout the day, since they can act for many hours. They contribute to high cortisol levels in the evening, which give your body the wrong message.
- Early morning awakening, around 3 or 4 A.M., often is a reflection of elevated cortisol levels, a sign of stress. Blood sugar may

dip, too. Consider taking the adrenal-support supplements (adaptogens) and modifying your lifestyle. A light protein snack at bedtime may also be helpful in maintaining blood-sugar levels.

- Exercise in the evening, which helps burn up the stress hormones of the day, but not within two hours before going to bed. Late-night exercise can be too stimulating.

- Don't eat late. You need to leave at least two hours between dinner and bedtime. Exception: protein snack for low blood-sugar problems.

- Do something relaxing before bed. This could be listening to music. Some meditative, repetitive music at a very low volume may help you fall asleep. If this works for you, the music may soon act as a trigger. Others prefer silence.

- Avoid stressful inputs just before bedtime. This includes the news and violent TV programs or movies.

- If you wake up in the early hours of the morning and sleep lightly in the morning, you may be serotonin-deficient, so try 500–2,000 mg of L-tryptophan, or 50–200 mg of 5-HTP, one hour before bedtime.

- If necessary, try 60–250 mg of kavalactones from kava. Do not exceed 250 mg a day. Or take 100–300 mg of valerian (with or without L-trytophan or 5-HTP). If combined, lower the doses of each product. There are excellent combination formulas available that also may include California poppy, skullcap, hops, passionflower, and/or reishi mushroom.

Part Four

NATURAL HIGHS
AT A GLANCE

22

Top Tips

In the Top Tips that follow, we give you instant programs to chill out, get an energy boost, improve your mood, sharpen your mind, and/or feel connected. As well as following these highly effective action plans, you also need to:

Follow the "Natural High Basics" and supplement guidelines in Chapter 3. If applicable, break your dependency to stimulants, cigarettes, drugs, and/or alcohol (see Chapter 9). Make sure you're not holding on to any unresolved emotions. If you are even a little bit upset with your mate, for example, a few words of clarification can go a long way toward domestic peace, and even bliss. If you are retaining work-related upsets, again, clear them either with the person involved, internally, or in a discussion with your partner, a friend, or whomever you can get to listen (and, preferably, empathize). Clinging to negative emotions is an energy and mood drain, while expressing them helps to dissipate the charge, allowing more energy for positive pursuits and for feeling high.

The supplement recommendations may seem overwhelming, but don't worry: You don't have to make all these decisions yourself. There are excellent combination formulas available that do that for you, with herbs and other supplements that work together synergistically in just the right proportion. (See Resources.)

Now on with the Top Tips!

Top Tips for a Natural Chill Out

If you come home from a hard day's work feeling stressed and in need of chilling out, here's what to do:

- Take any of the following natural "chillers," based on your own experimentation. The suggested doses are guidelines only, since each of us has a unique biochemical makeup. You can start with 60–75 mg of kava (kavalactones) daily, increasing to two to three times daily, if that's what works for you. If you still don't feel relaxed, try, or add, any of the following, preferably one at a time to gauge your response. (If you do end up taking them all, reduce the dose of each by one-half, or take a combination formula.) Take about 60 mg of valerian, 100 mg of hops, 100 mg of passionflower, 500 mg of GABA, or 500 mg of taurine.
- Do a vital energy exercise—yoga, t'ai chi, or any form of movement or dance.
- Take a bath with essential oils of lavender, orange, marjoram, and/or chamomile dispersed in the water.
- Meditate, listen to biofeedback tapes, or do a breathing exercise.
- Listen to relaxing music.
- Have someone give you a massage, or give yourself one.
- Light your room with candles and/or blue or turquoise light.
- Have sex.
- Take a nap if you need one.

Top Tips for a Natural Energy Boost

If your "get up and go" has "got up and went" and you need a natural energy boost, here's what to do:

- Take any of the following energy boosters, based on your own experimentation. The suggested doses are guidelines only, since each of us has a unique biochemical makeup. You can start with 400 mg of Siberian ginseng, 500 mg of licorice, and 100 mg of pantothenic acid. (The last two are more for adrenal support than actual energy.) Or take either 500 mg of the amino acid tyrosine *or* 500 mg of DLPA. Depending on your response, you can add in any or all of the following to create your own personal energy formula, preferably one at a time to gauge your response. This can differ from day to day, too, depending on how you are feeling. If you do end up taking them all, reduce the dose of each accordingly, about one-third to one-half. Take about 100 mg of Asian or American ginseng, 300 mg of ashwaganda, 3,000 mg of reishi mushroom, 100 mg of rhodiola, 100–250 mg of DLPA, *or* 100–250 mg of tyrosine.
- Take a bath with essential oils of lemon, eucalyptus, cinnamon, or peppermint dispersed in the water, or scent your room with them.
- Do aerobic exercise.
- Do a vital energy exercise—yoga, t'ai chi, Psychocalisthenics, or any form of movement or dance.
- Listen to stimulating music and boogie to the beat.
- Maximize the light in your room with natural daylight or full-spectrum lighting.

Top Tips for a Natural Mood Lift

If you're feeling low and need to perk up to get back on track, here's what to do:

- Take the following mood boosters: 100 mg of vitamin B_5, 20 mg of vitamin B_6, 10 mcg of vitamin B_{12}, and 400 mcg of folic acid; 50 mg of 5-HTP (increase gradually to 200 mg) *or* 900 mg of St. John's wort. (Remember, St. John's wort may take a few days or even a few weeks to kick in, but it's worth the wait.) Use caution in combining 5-HTP and St. John's wort (serotonin syndrome).

Your mood-boosting formula can also include some or all of the following (add one new product at a time to see how you respond): 50 mg of 5-HTP, 300 mg of St. John's wort, 500 mg of tyrosine, 500 mg of DLPA, 200 mg of SAMe *or* 600 mg of TMG, and 40 mg of vitamin B_3 (niacin).

- Do some aerobic exercise and/or a vital energy exercise—yoga, t'ai chi, or dance.
- Do the Light Exercise (see page 275).
- Listen to inspiring music, the kind that goes right to your heart and soul.
- Take a bath with essential oils of bergamot, geranium, petitgrain, or neroli dispersed in the water, or scent your room with them.
- Maximize the light in your room with natural daylight or full-spectrum lighting.

Top Tips for a Natural Mind Enhancement

If your razor-sharp intellect is blunted and your memory is failing you, here's what to do for that extra mental edge:

- Take a B-complex supplement that provides 50 mg each of vitamins B_3, B_5, B_6, and B_{12}, and 400 mcg of folic acid (in addition to what's in your multivitamin); also take 1,000 mg of EPA/DHA, *or* eat fish three times a week.

  Your mind-boosting formula can contain any or all of the following. Experiment with the individual products to get your own special mix. Start with 60 mg of ginkgo. Then add in 200 mg of phosphatidyl choline, 200 mg of DMAE, 10 mg of vinpocetine, and 50 mg of phosphatidylserine. These doses are acceptable in a combined formula, but, again, use your own response as the measure.

- Do some aerobic exercise to oxygenate your brain, raise endorphins, and, as an added bonus, burn some fat.
- Take a bath with essential oils of lemon, eucalyptus, cinnamon, or peppermint dispersed in the water, or scent your room with them.

- Listen to stimulating music.
- Maximize the light in your room with natural daylight or full-spectrum lighting.

Top Tips for Getting Connected Naturally

If you're feeling disconnected and you've lost your sparkle, here's how to get reconnected and back in the flow:

- Take the following "connectors." Start with kava, the heart and social opener, at a dose of 60–75 mg of kavalactones in a standardized extract. Always take a B-complex supplement providing 50 mg of each of the vitamins B_3, B_5, B_6, and B_{12}, and 400 mcg of folic acid (in addition to the amount in your multivitamin). Add 200 mg of SAMe (taken separately), then 50 mg of 5-HTP. Your "connector nutrient" formula can include 50 mg of 5-HTP, 200 mg of SAMe *or* 600 mg of TMG, 60–75 mg of kava, and 100 mg of sceletium.
- Listen to heart- and soul-inspiring music
- Do a vital energy exercise—yoga, t'ai chi, Psychocalisthenics, or any form of movement or dance.
- Meditate or listen to biofeedback tapes.
- Have someone give you a massage, or give yourself one.
- Take a bath with essential oil of lavender dispersed in the water, or scent your room with it.
- Light your room with candles or violet, magenta, or blue light.

23

A to Z of Natural Highs

Acetyl-L-carnitine

• MIND AND MEMORY BOOSTER

How it works: Fuel for the brain; helps make acetylcholine; acts as an antioxidant.
Positive effects: Improves mood and mental performance.
Cautions: Not recommended for those with diabetes, liver disease, or kidney disease.
Dosage: 250–1,500 mg daily, between meals.

Ashwaganda *(Withania somnifera)*

• ADAPTOGEN
• ENERGIZER

How it works: Acts as an adaptogen; stabilizes cortisol levels; acetylcholine enhancer.

Positive effects: Energizes and calms; reduces high cortisol levels; enhances libido, memory, and cognition.

Cautions: None.

Dosage: 300 mg two to three times daily.

B Vitamins

- ENERGIZERS
- MOOD ENHANCERS
- MIND AND MEMORY BOOSTERS
- CONNECTORS

How they work: Turn glucose into energy in neurons; cofactors for making neurotransmitters; help transport oxygen; protect the brain from toxins and oxidants; vital for enzymes that control the chemistry of connection; act as methyl group donors and acceptors.

Positive effects: Raise IQ; improve energy, memory, mood, and concentration; help to prevent the unpleasant hallucinations experienced in some types of schizophrenia.

Cautions: None when taken in sensible doses. Excess B_3 and B_6 (above 1,000 mg a day) can have adverse effects. B_3 as niacin acts as a vasodilator, improving circulation and causing flushing at doses above 50 mg.

Dosage: 20–100 mg daily of each of the following: B_1, B_2, B_3, and B_6; 50–500 mg of B_5; 10–1,000 mcg of B_{12}; 400–800 mcg of folic acid.

Choline

- MIND AND MEMORY BOOSTER

How it works: Precursor for the neurotransmitter acetylcholine; part of the structure of neuronal membranes.

Positive effects: More alert, clear-headed, better memory and concentration; improved brain development during pregnancy in rats.

Cautions: None.

Dosage: (Daily) 5–10 g (approximately 1 tablespoon) of lecithin, *or* 2.5–5 g (a heaping tablespoon) of hi-phosphatidylcholine lecithin, *or* 1–2 g of phosphatidyl choline, *or* 500 mg–2 g of choline chloride (fishy smelling); and 500–1,000 mg of citicholine and 500–1,500 mg of alpha-GPC.

Coenzyme Q_{10} (CoQ_{10})

- ENERGIZER

How it works: Stimulates cellular production of energy; antioxidant.

Positive effects: Is a good antioxidant; enhances energy and endurance; helps repair receding gums.

Cautions: None.

Dosage: 30–300 mg daily, depending on individual requirements.

DHA (an omega-3 fat)

- MOOD ENHANCER
- MIND AND MEMORY BOOSTER

How it works: Building material for neuronal membranes and neurotransmitter receptor sites; increases acetylcholine and serotonin levels.

Positive effects: Improves learning, memory, and mood in depression, manic depression, dyslexia, and dyspraxia.

Cautions: DHA helps reduce blood clotting; therefore, high doses should not be taken if you are on blood-thinning medication.

Dosage: 250–1,000 mg a day as a fish oil supplement, or eat 3 ounces of fatty fish three times a week.

DMAE

- MIND AND MEMORY BOOSTER

How it works: Precursor for choline that crosses readily into the brain, thereby helping to make acetylcholine. May also enhance dopamine activity.

Positive effects: Increases alertness; improves concentration; reduces anxiety; improves learning and attention span; normalizes brain-wave patterns.

Cautions: Too much can overstimulate and is therefore not recommended for those diagnosed with schizophrenia, mania, or epilepsy. Lower the dosage if you experience insomnia.

Dosage: 100–300 mg daily, taken in the morning or midday, not in the evening.

EPA (an omega-3 fat)

- MOOD ENHANCER
- MIND AND MEMORY BOOSTER

How it works: Precursor for prostaglandins, chemicals that influence mood and behavior and probably affect neurotransmitter balance.

Positive effects: Helps restore normal mood in bipolar illness. May also affect memory.

Cautions: EPA helps reduce blood clotting. High doses should not be taken if you are on blood-thinning medication.

Dosage: 500–1,000 mg a day as a fish oil supplement, or eat 3 ounces of fatty fish three times a week. Take with 400 IU of vitamin E daily as an antioxidant.

GABA

- STRESS BUSTER

How it works: Calming neurotransmitter; enhances GABA activity, which counteracts stress hormones.
Positive effect: Reduces anxiety, insomnia, and tension.
Cautions: Can cause nausea and vomiting at high doses.
Dosage: 250–500 mg twice daily after meals.

Ginkgo Biloba

- MIND AND MEMORY BOOSTER

How it works: Improves circulation; acts as an antioxidant.
Positive effects: Improves mood, memory, concentration, and energy.
Cautions: Blood thinner: use with caution if taking blood-thinning medication. Rare side effects of headaches, nausea, or nosebleeds have been reported at high doses.
Dosage: 120–240 mg a day of a standardized extract providing 24 percent flavonoids, taken in two divided doses (60–120 mg twice daily).

Ginseng—Siberian, Asian, and American

- ENERGIZERS
- ADAPTOGEN

How they work: Adaptogens; support the adrenal glands.
Positive effects: Enhance the body's response to stress; decrease feelings of anxiety and stress; increase immediate energy (stimulants); restore vitality, energy, and endurance over time (tonics); increase mental and physical performance.
Cautions: None for Siberian ginseng. For Asian ginseng, possible men-

strual abnormalities and breast tenderness. Overuse can cause overstimulation, including insomnia in sensitive individuals. Take a one-month
break after taking ginseng for three months.

Dosage: 200–400 mg daily of Siberian ginseng; *or* 100–200 mg daily of
Asian or American ginseng (standardized extract containing 4 to 7 percent ginsenosides).

Glutamine

- STRESS BUSTER
- ENERGIZER
- MIND AND MEMORY BOOSTER

How it works: Fuel for brain cells; helps build and balance neurotransmitters.

Positive effects: Improves both mental energy and relaxation; reduces addiction; stabilizes blood sugar; promotes memory.

Cautions: Rare reports of headaches at high doses.

Dosage: 2,000–5,000 mg daily between meals.

Green Tea

- STRESS BUSTER
- ENERGIZER

How it works: Contains potent antioxidants, theanine, and caffeine.

Positive effects: Lowers cholesterol and blood pressure; increases HDL,
the so-called "good" cholesterol; thins the blood; reduces risk of heart
attack, stroke, and cancer; enhances immune function; prevents dental
caries and hypertension; aids weight loss by encouraging the body to
burn fat; produces a state of alert relaxation.

Cautions: Contains caffeine.

Dosage: 1–2 cups a day.

5-HTP. *See* Tryptophan and 5-HTP.

Kava

- STRESS BUSTER
- CONNECTOR

How it works: Calms the limbic system, the emotional center of the brain; relaxes muscles, likely through an indirect action on GABA receptors; appears to enhance GABA activity, the relaxing neurotransmitter that also modulates dopamine, adrenaline, and noradrenaline. (There is still much that is unknown about its effects on the brain.)

Positive effects: Relaxes the mind, emotions, and muscles, making it useful for headaches, backaches, and other tension; promotes good sleep; reduces excessive mental chatter; increases mental focus; heightens sensory perception; expands overall awareness; promotes well-being, connection, and empathy. No habituation, tolerance, addiction, or hangover is associated with kava.

Cautions: Do not drive or operate heavy machinery after use. Do not mix with alcohol, as the two substances seem to potentiate each other. Do not take while using benzodiazepine tranquilizers. Do not take if you have impaired liver function.

Dosage: As a relaxant, 60–75 mg of kavalactones two to three times daily. As a bedtime sedative, take 60–250 mg.

Licorice

- ADAPTOGEN
- ENERGIZER

How it works: Adaptogen; prevents the breakdown of cortisol, thereby raising cortisol levels.
Positive effects: Improves adrenal function, including raising low blood pressure.
Cautions: Can raise blood pressure in susceptible individuals. Not recommended for those with raised cortisol levels.
Dosage: 500 mg twice a day, morning and midday, not in the evening.

NADH

- ENERGIZER

How it works: Stimulates cellular production of the neurotransmitters dopamine, noradrenaline, and serotonin.
Positive effects: It is a good antioxidant; improves mental clarity, cellular memory, alertness, and concentration; enhances energy and athletic endurance.
Cautions: None.
Dosage: 2.5–10 mg daily, depending on individual requirements.

DL-phenylalanine (DLPA)

- ENERGIZER
- MOOD ENHANCER

How it works: Precursor for tyrosine, which converts to dopamine, adrenaline, and noradrenaline.

Positive effects: Enhances mood; promotes energy; relieves pain; controls appetite.

Cautions: Can be too stimulating, generating anxiety, high blood pressure, and/or insomnia; should not be taken by phenylketonurics. Not recommended for those with a history of mania or other types of mental illness.

Dosage: 500–1,000 mg daily before morning meal. Can be repeated later in the day, but not too close to bedtime. Add 25–50 mg of vitamin B_6 and 500 mg of vitamin C daily to enhance its conversion to tyrosine.

Phosphatidylserine

- MIND AND MEMORY BOOSTER

How it works: Building material for neuronal membranes and neurotransmitter receptor sites.

Positive effects: Improves mood, memory, stress resistance, learning, and concentration.

Cautions: None.

Dosage: 100–300 mg daily.

Pyroglutamate

- MIND AND MEMORY BOOSTER

How it works: Increases acetylcholine production and improves reception.

Positive effects: Improves memory, cognitive function, concentration, coordination, and reaction time; improves communication between the right and left hemispheres of the brain.

Cautions: None.

Dosage: 400–1,000 mg daily.

Reishi Mushroom

- ADAPTOGEN
- ENERGIZER

How it works: Adaptogen; stabilizes adrenal hormones.
Positive effects: Both calms and energizes.
Cautions: None.
Dosage: In tincture form (20 percent), 10 ml three times a day; as tablets, 1,000 mg, one to three tablets three times a day.

Rhodiola

- ENERGIZER

How it works: Adaptogen; stabilizes adrenal hormones; promotes serotonin production.
Positive effects: Improves concentration, stress resistance, physical performance, and mood; boosts immunity.
Cautions: None.
Dosage: 100 mg of standardized extract two to three times daily with meals.

SAMe and TMG

- MOOD ENHANCERS
- CONNECTORS

How they work: Naturally occurring molecules, donate methyl groups in manufacture of neurotransmitters and DNA. They therefore act as catalysts for producing a wide range of key brain chemicals, including DMT, serotonin, dopamine, and noradrenaline. SAMe is produced from the amino acid methionine. Also important in liver detoxification.

Positive effects: Enhance neurotransmitter activity; act as natural antide-pressants, stimulants, and mood enhancers; generally improve energy, mental clarity, emotional balance, and mood, promoting natural connection.

Cautions: In some people, higher doses of SAMe have been known to induce nausea. Taking SAMe with food reduces this possibility but somewhat decreases its potency. Very high doses may lead to irritability, anxiety, and insomnia. SAMe's antidepressant activity may lead to the manic phase in individuals with bipolar disorder (manic depression), so monitor carefully.

Dosage: As a connector, 200–800 mg of SAMe between meals to promote absorption, *or* 500–3,000 mg of TMG (trimethyl glycine) metabolite. For depression, 200 mg of SAMe twice daily between meals, increasing gradually to a maximum of 1,600 mg daily, if needed, *or* 250–500 mg once or twice daily.

Sceletium

* MOOD ENHANCER
* CONNECTOR

How it works: Appears to enhance activity of serotonin, the mood-enhancing neurotransmitter; helps to balance dopamine, adrenaline, and noradrenaline. (There is still much that is unknown about its effects on the brain.)

Positive effects: Lessens depression, tension, and anxiety; promotes a sense of connection; associated with insights, heightened sensory perception, and improved meditation; also reduces addictive cravings.

Cautions: In very large doses it can have euphoric effects, followed by sedation. Sceletium has not been researched sufficiently to recommend its use during pregnancy or nursing. No reported toxicity. However, we recommend not taking it with antidepressants. If combined with large amounts of tryptophan or 5-HTP, there is the possibility of serotonin syndrome—headache, an increase in body temperature, and heavy sweating. Stop taking it and seek medical advice if this occurs.

Dosage: As a mood enhancer, 50–100 mg daily; as a connector, 100–200 mg daily.

St. John's Wort

• MOOD ENHANCER

How it works: Appears to inhibit reuptake of the neurotransmitters serotonin, norepinephrine, and dopamine; enhances GABA activity.

Positive effects: Enhances mood; acts as an antidepressant; combats anxiety in most people; helps regulate sleep.

Cautions: May cause allergic reactions, rashes, gastrointestinal problems,
or sun sensitivity in susceptible individuals. Can cause anxiety or insomnia if taken too close to bedtime. Can reduce the potency of protease
inhibitors (taken as treatment for AIDS) or cyclosporin (an immunosuppressant taken by organ transplant patients), digoxin (heart medication), or even birth control pills. St. John's wort has not been researched
sufficiently to recommend it for use during pregnancy or nursing. If
combined with 5-HTP, there's the possibility of serotonin syndrome—
headache, an increase in body temperature, and heavy sweating. Seek
medical help if this occurs.

Dosage: 300 mg daily of an extract of 0.3 percent hypericin, starting with
one to two capsules or tablets in the morning with breakfast. If there is
no change in mood after a week, add a third dose at lunch, for a total of
900 mg daily. You can also take it as two doses of 450 mg each, or take
your entire daily dose in the morning, since the herb stays in the body
for approximately 24 hours before being broken down.

Taurine

• STRESS BUSTER

How it works: Enhances the activity of GABA, the calming neurotransmitter.

Positive effects: Reduces anxiety, irritability, insomnia, migraine, alcoholism,
obsessions, and depression.

Cautions: None reported.

Dosage: 250–500 mg twice daily, between meals.

Tryptophan and 5-HTP

- MOOD ENHANCERS
- CONNECTORS

How they work: Precursors for the neurotransmitter serotonin and some tryptamines. L-tryptophan is a precursor to 5-HTP and can also be diverted to produce niacin (vitamin B$_3$).

Positive effects: Elevate mood; promote relaxation, deep sleep, healthy sleep-wake patterns, emotional stability, dreaming, and creative imagination.

Cautions: Nausea and gastrointestinal problems in high doses. Due to the theoretical risk of serotonin syndrome, it is not advisable to take both 5-HTP and SSRI antidepressants except under medical guidance.

Dosage: For depression or insomnia, take 100–300 mg daily of 5-HTP, *or* take 1,000–3,000 mg daily of L-tryptophan. As a mood enhancer or natural connector, take 100 mg daily of 5-HTP, preferably as 50 mg twice daily; *or* take 1,000 mg of L-tryptophan. Best absorbed away from protein, with a carbohydrate snack, such as a piece of fruit or fruit juice, and with B vitamins.

Tyrosine

- ENERGIZER
- MOOD ENHANCER

How it works: Precursor to the stimulating neurotransmitters dopamine, adrenaline, noradrenaline, and the thyroid hormone, thyroxine.

Positive effects: Enhances mood; promotes energy and motivation; supports healthy thyroid function.

Cautions: Hypertension in those susceptible. Should not be taken by phenylketonurics, those with melanomas, or pregnant or nursing women. Not recommended for those with a history of mania, unless under a doctor's care.

Dosage: 100–1,000 mg daily before morning meal to prevent competition from other amino acids. Can be repeated in mid-afternoon.

Valerian

• STRESS BUSTER

How it works: Enhances GABA activity.
Positive effects: Reduces anxiety, insomnia, and tension.
Cautions: Potentiates sedative drugs, including muscle relaxants and anti-histamines; can interact with alcohol.
Dosage: As a relaxant, 50–100 mg two to three times daily; as a bedtime sedative, 100–300 mg about 45 minutes before bedtime.

Vinpocetine

• MIND AND MEMORY BOOSTER

How it works: Improves blood flow and circulation to the brain.
Positive effects: Improves cognitive performance; potentially helpful in epilepsy.
Cautions: None reported.
Dosage: 10–40 mg a day.

Glossary

acetylcholine A stimulating neurotransmitter associated with memory, mental alertness, learning ability, and concentration. Acetylcholine deficiency can lead to memory loss, depression, mood disorders, and possibly even Alzheimer's disease. It is also the neurotransmitter at all nerve-muscle cell junctions that allows skeletal muscles to contract, controlling movement, coordination, and muscle tone.

addiction A pattern of compulsive consumption of a substance, accompanied by a need for increased doses over time to maintain the same effect (tolerance) or to avoid symptoms of "withdrawal."

adrenaline (also called epinephrine) A stimulating neurotransmitter associated with motivation, drive, energy, stimulation, and the stress response. Produced by the adrenal glands, it is also classified as a hormone, which is a chemical messenger produced by the glands of the endocrine system.

amino acid A building block of protein. Plants and animals assemble amino acids to make proteins that form different substances such as hormones, neurotransmitters, and building materials for the body, such as muscle or skin.

amphetamine A stimulant drug that blocks neurons' re-absorption of the neurotransmitters noradrenaline and dopamine and also triggers their release. Often prescribed to treat attention deficit disorder (ADD and ADHD).

Glossary

antioxidants A family of nutrients with the ability to bind with and render harmless the oxidants or free radicals that cause cell damage, disease, and aging. These include vitamins A, C, and E; the minerals zinc and selenium; plus glutathione and cysteine, and plant-based antioxidants such as anthocyanidins (found in berries, grapes, and similar fruits).

dendrites Branches that connect nerve cells (neurons) with one another. A neuron can have up to 20,000 dendrites networking with other neurons.

dopamine A stimulating neurotransmitter associated with pleasure, alertness, concentration, and euphoria. Adrenaline and noradrenaline are both made from dopamine.

downregulation The shutting down of neurotransmitter receptor sites as a consequence of over-stimulation, resulting in the need for increased doses of a substance over time to maintain the same effect (tolerance).

endorphins A popular term for substances known as "opiate peptides," which include enkephalins and dynorphins. These are associated with pleasure, orgasm, euphoria, and pain relief. Endorphins are the brain's own natural opiates: They bind to a specific opiate receptor, reducing pain and promoting mild euphoria, such as "runner's high."

free radicals Highly reactive molecules formed by normal metabolic oxidative reactions, as well as by chemicals that we ingest and inhale from our environment. They bind to and destroy cells that lack a good supply of protective antioxidants.

GABA (gamma-amino-butyric acid) An inhibitory neurotransmitter, associated with relaxation. It has a quieting or dampening effect on the central nervous system and controls the release of dopamine in the reward center of the brain.

monoamine oxidase inhibitor (MAOI) A type of antidepressant drug that inhibits the enzyme monoamine oxidase, which breaks down neurotransmitters. Therefore, MAOI has the effect of keeping more neurotransmitters in action.

myelin sheath The insulating layer or membrane around a nerve cell (neuron), made largely out of phospholipids and fatty acids.

neuron Nerve cells that form the "road map" of our nervous system. They exist throughout the body but are highly concentrated in the brain.

neurotransmitter A molecule capable of stimulating a neuron. Neurotransmitters are therefore the nervous system's chemicals of communication and are usually made out of amino acids.

Glossary

nootropic Pronounced "no-a-tropic," it refers to the smart drugs that "enhance cognition." Some nootropics block the breakdown of neurotransmitters; others mimic or improve the action of neurotransmitters; and still others are manufactured versions of hormones that influence brain function.

phospholipid A type of semi-essential nutrient—made by the body and required in the diet for optimal health—that is part of the membrane (myelin sheath) of neurons. Two types of phospholipids, phosphatidyl choline and phosphatidyl serine, are especially important for optimal health and brain function.

receptor site The docking port for neurotransmitters, embedded in the membrane of a neuron. Receptor sites are specific for different kinds of neurotransmitters.

selective serotonin re-uptake inhibitor (SSRI) A type of antidepressant drug that inhibits the neurotransmitter serotonin being re-uptaken into the neuron from which it was released, hence keeping more serotonin in action.

serotonin A neurotransmitter associated with mood, sleep patterns, dreaming, and visions. It influences many physiological functions, including blood pressure, digestion, body temperature, and pain sensation. Serotonin also affects mood as well as circadian rhythm, the body's response to the cycles of day and night.

synapse The gap between the dendrite and the neuron to which the dendrite connects. Neurotransmitters move from one neuron to another across this gap.

tolerance The need for increased doses of a substance over time to maintain the same effect as a result of "downregulation."

upregulation The opening up of neurotransmitter receptor sites as a consequence of under-stimulation, such as withdrawal from an addictive substance, resulting in less need for external stimulants.

withdrawal The occurrence of unpleasant symptoms upon the discontinuation of the use of an addictive substance, which disappear when the substance is reinstated.

References

CHAPTER 2: HOW YOUR BRAIN KEEPS YOU HIGH

Smith, K. A., et al. "Relapse of depression after rapid depletion of tryptophan." *Lancet* 349: 915–19.

CHAPTER 3: NATURAL HIGH BASICS

Benton, D. "Effect of vitamin and mineral supplementation on intelligence of a sample of school children." *Lancet* 1 (1988): 140–44.
Oakley, G. P. "Eat right and take a multivitamin." *New England Journal of Medicine* (9 Apr. 1998): 1060–61.

CHAPTER 4: STRESS BUSTERS

Julien, R. *A Primer of Drug Action.* New York: Freeman and Co., 1998, p. 340.
Lader, M. "Benzodiazepines—the opiate of the masses?" *Neuroscience* 3 (1978): 159–65.

Lemert, E. M. "Secular use of kava in Tonga." *Quarterly Journal of Studies on Alcohol* 18 (1967): 328–41.

Lindenberg, D., et al. "Kava in comparison with oxazepam in anxiety disorders: a double-blind study of clinical effectiveness." *Fortschr Med* 108 (1990): 49–50.

Litovitz, T. L., et al. 1999 annual report of the American Association of Poison Control Center's Toxic Exposure Surveillance System. *American Journal of Emergency Medicine* 18(5) (Sept. 2000): 517–74.

Münte, T. F., H. J. Heinze, M. Matzke, and J. Steitz. "Effects of oxazepam and an extract of kava root *(Piper methysticum)* on event-related potentials in a word-recognition task." *Neuropsychobiology* 27(1) (1993): 46–53.

Office of National Drug Control Policy. "What America's users spend on illegal drugs, 1988–1998."

Pope, H. G., et al. "Neuropsychological performance in long-term cannabis users." *Archives of General Psychiatry* 58 (Oct. 2001).

Shiah, I. S., and N. Yatham. "GABA functions in mood disorders: an update and critical review." *Nature Life Sciences* 63(15) (1998): 1289–1303.

Theroux, P. *The Happy Isles of Oceania.* New York: Putnam, 1992, p. 42.

Volz, H. P., and M. Kieser. "Kava-kava extract WS 1490 versus placebo in anxiety disorders—a randomized placebo-controlled 25-week outpatient trial." *Pharmacopsychiatry* 30 (1997): 1–5.

Williams, R. "Classification, etiology, and considerations of outcome in acute liver failure." *Semin. Liver Dis.* 16(4) (Nov. 1996): 343–38.

Woelk, H., et al. "Double-blind study: kava extract versus benzodiazepines in treatment of patients suffering from anxiety." *Z Allg Med* 69 (1993): 271–77.

CHAPTER 5: ENERGIZERS

Astrup, A. "The effect of ephedrine/caffeine mixture on energy expenditure and body composition in obese women." *Metabolism* 41(7) (1992): 686–88.

Balagot, R. C. "Analgesia in mice and humans by D-phenylalanine: relation to inhibition of enkephalin degradation and enkephalin levels." *Advances in Pain Research and Therapy* 5 (1983): 289–92.

Beckmann, H., et al. "DL-phenylalanine versus imipramine: a double-blind controlled study." *Archives of Psychiatric Diseases* 227 (1979): 49–58.

Blumenthal, M., and P. King. "Ma huang: ancient herb, modern medicine, regulatory dilemma: a review of the botany, chemistry, medicinal uses, safety concerns and legal status of ephedra and its alkaloids." *HerbalGram* 134 (1995): 22–57.

Brekman, I. I., and I. V. Dardymov. "New substances of plant origin which increase nonspecific resistance." *Annual Review of Pharmacology and Toxicology* 9 (1969): 419–30.

References

Budd, K. "Use of D-phenylalanine, an enkephalinase inhibitor, in the treatment of intractable pain." *Advances in Pain Research and Therapy* 5 (1983): 305–8.

Carper, J. *Your Miracle Brain*. New York: HarperCollins, 2000.

Deijen, J. B., et al. "Tyrosine improves cognitive performance and reduces blood pressure in cadets." *Brain Research Bulletin* 48(2) (1999): 203–9.

Gilliland, K., and D. Andress. "Ad lib caffeine consumption, symptoms of caffeinism, and academic performance." *American Journal of Psychiatry* 138(4) (1981): 512–14.

James, J. "Acute and chronic effects of caffeine on performance, mood, headache, and sleep." *Neuropsychobiology* 38 (1998): 32–42.

Mason, R. *200 mg of Zen: Alternative and Complementary Therapies*. Larchmont, NY: Mary Ann Liebert, Inc., 2001.

Ploss, E. "Panax ginseng," *Kooperation Phytopharmaka*, Cologne (1988); and Sonnenborn, U., and Y. Proppert. "Panax ginseng." *Z. Phytotherapie* 11 (1990): 35–49. Both papers quoted in V. Schultz, et al. *Rational Phytotherapy*, New York: Springer (1998): 272.

Sabelli, H. C., et al. "Clinical studies on the phenylethylamine hypothesis of affective disorder." *Journal of Clinical Psychiatry* 47 (1986): 66–70.

Science news report (11 Feb. 2000).

CHAPTER 6: MOOD ENHANCERS

Bressa, G. M. "S-adenosyl-methionine as antidepressant: meta-analysis of clinical studies." *Acta Neurologica Scandanavian Supplement* 154 (1994): 7–14.

Dubini, A., et al. "Do noradrenaline and serotonin differentially affect social motivation and behavior?" *European Neuropsychopharmacology* 7(1) (1997): S49–55.

Eccleston, D. "L-tryptophan and depressive illness." *Psychiatric Bulletin* 17 (1993): 223–34.

Godfrey, P. S., et al. "Enhancement of recovery from psychiatric illness by methylfolate." *Lancet* 336 (1990): 392–95.

Linde, K., et al. "St. John's wort for depression: an overview and meta-analysis of randomised clinical trials." *British Medical Journal* 313(7052) (1996): 253–58.

Miller, A. "St. John's wort (*Hypericum perforatum*): clinical effects on depression." *Alternative Medicine Review* 3(1) (1998): 18–26.

Poldinger, W., et al. "A functional-dimensional approach to depression: serotonin deficiency and target syndrome in a comparison of 5-hydroxytryptophan and fluvoxamine." *Psychopathology* 24 (1991): 53–81.

Smith, K. A., et al. "Relapse of depression after rapid depletion of tryptophan." *Lancet* 349 (1997): 915–19.

Vorbach, E. U., et al. "Efficacy and tolerability of St. John's wort extract LI 160 vs. imipramine in patients with severe depressive episodes according to ICD-10." *Pharmacopsychiatry* 30(2) (1997): 81–85.

CHAPTER 7: MIND AND MEMORY BOOSTERS

Allard, M. "Treatment of old-age disorders with ginkgo biloba extract." *La Presse Medicale* 15(31) (1995): 1540.

Alvarez, X. A., et al. "Citicholine improves memory performance in elderly subjects." Methods and findings in *Experimental and Clinical Pharmacology* 19(30) (Apr. 1997): 20–210.

Bartus, R. T., et al. "Profound effects of combining choline and piracetam on memory enhancement and cholinergic function in aged rats." *Neurobiology of Ageing* 2 (1981): 105–11.

Benton, D., and G. Roberts. "Effect of vitamin and mineral supplementation on intelligence of a sample of schoolchildren." *Lancet* 1 (1988): 140–44.

Benton, D., et al. "The impact of long-term vitamin supplementation on cognitive functioning." *Psychopharmacology* 117 (1995): 298–305.

Catayud, M., et al. "Effects of CDP-choline on the recovery of patients with head injury." *Journal of the Neurological Sciences* 103 (July 1991): S15–18.

Crook, T., et al. "Effects of phosphatidyl serine in age-associated memory impairment." *Neurology* 41(5) (1991): 644–49.

Dean, W., J. Morgenthaler, and S. Fowkes. (Cases published in) *Smart Drugs 2: The Next Generation*. Petaluma, CA: Smart Publications, 1993.

Dimpfel, W., et al. "Source density analysis of functional topographical EEG: monitoring of cognitive drug action." *European Journal of Medical Research* 1(6) (19 Mar. 1996): 283–90.

Ferris, S., et al. "Combination of choline/piracetam in the treatment of senile dementia." *Psychopharmacology Bulletin* 18 (1982): 94–98.

Funfgeld, E. "A natural and broad spectrum nootropic substance for treatment of SDAT—the ginkgo biloba extract." *Progress in Clinical and Biological Research* 317 (1989): 1247–60.

Hibbeln, J. R. "Fish consumption and major depression." *Lancet* 351 (1998): 1213.

Hindmarch, I. "Activity of ginkgo biloba extract on short-term memory." *La Presse Medicale* 15(31) (1995): 1562–92.

Hindmarch, I., et al. "Efficacy and tolerance of vinpocetine in ambulant patients suffering from mild to moderate organic psychosyndromes." *International Clinical Psychopharmacology* 6(1) (1991): 31–43.

Kleijnen, J., and P. Knipschild. "Ginkgo biloba." *Lancet* 340(8828) (1992): 1136–39.

Le Bars, P. L. "A placebo-controlled, double-blind, randomized trial on an extract of ginkgo biloba for dementia." *Journal of the American Medical Association* 278(16) (1997): 1327–32.

Loriaux, S., et al. "The effects of nicotinic acid (niacin) and xanthinol nicotinate on human memory in different categories of age. A double-blind study." *Psychopharmacology* 87 (1985): 390–95.

Lupien, S. "Longitudinal increase in cortisol during human aging, hippocampal atrophy and memory deficits." *Nature Neuroscience* 1(1) (May 1998): 69–73.

Meck, W. H., et al. "Characterization of the facilitative effects of perinatal choline supplementation on timing and temporal memory." *Neuroreport* 8(13) (Dec. 1997): 2831–35.

Pearson, D., and S. Shaw. *Life Extension: A Practical Scientific Approach.* New York: Warner Books, 1982.

Pyapali, G., et al. "Prenatal dietary choline supplementation." *Journal of Neurophysiology* 79(4) (1998): 1790–96.

Sahelian, R. *Mind Boosters.* New York: St. Martin's Press, 2000, p. 185.

Sapolsky, R. M. "Why stress is bad for your brain." *Science* 273(5276) (1996): 749–50.

Shabert, J., et al. *The Ultimate Nutrient—Glutamine.* Garden City, NY: Avery Publishing, 1994.

Snowden, W. "Analysis of errors and omissions in IQ tests." *Personality and Individual Differences* 22(1) (1997): 131–34.

Stewart, J. W., et al. "Low B_6 levels in depressed patients." *Biological Psychiatry* 141 (1982): 271–72.

Stoll, A. L., et al. "Omega-3 fatty acids in bipolar disorder." *Archives of General Psychiatry* 56 (1999): 407.

Stordy, B. J. "Benefit of docosahexaenoic acid supplements of dark adaptation in dyslexics." *Lancet* 346 (1995): 385.

CHAPTER 8: MAKING THE CONNECTION

Cass, H. "SAMe—the master tuner supplement for the 21st century." *Total Health* 22(1). (Also on www.naturallyhigh.co.uk).

Cass, H., and T. McNally. *Kava: Nature's Answer to Stress, Anxiety and Insomnia.* Rockville, CA: Prima Publishing, 1998.

Doblin, R., et al. "Dr. Oscar Janiger's pioneering LSD research: a forty year follow-up." *Multidisciplinary Association for Psychedelic Studies Journal* 9(1) (1999). (Available on www.maps.org).

Dowling, G., et al. "'Eve' and 'ecstasy': a report of five deaths associated with the use of MDEA and MDMA." *Journal of the American Medical Association* 257 (1987): 1615–17.

Godfrey, P., et al. "Enhancement of recovery from psychiatric illness." *Lancet* 336 (1990): 392–95.

Greenberg, G. "The serotonin surprise." *Discover* 22(7) (2001): 68.

Harrington, R., et al. "Life-threatening interactions between HIV-1 protease inhibitors and the illicit drugs MDMA and gamma-hydroxybutyrate." *Archives of Internal Medicine* 159 (Oct. 1999): 2221–24.

Hatzidimitriou, G., U. D. McCann, and G. A. Ricaurte. "Altered serotonin innervation patterns in the forebrain of monkeys treated with MDMA seven years previously: factors influencing abnormal recovery." *Journal of Neuroscience* 19(12) (15 June 1999): 5096–107.

Hoffer, A., et al. "Treatment of schizophrenia with nicotinic acid and nicotinamide." *Journal of Clinical Experimental Psychopathology* 18 (1957): 131–58.

Lemert, E. "Secular use of kava in Tonga." *Quarterly Journal of Studies on Alcohol* 18 (1967): 328–41.

Manchanda, S., and M. Connolly. "Cerebral infarction in association with ecstasy abuse." *Postgraduate Medical Journal* 69 (1993): 874–79.

McCann, U. D., et al. "Positron emission tomographic evidence of MDMA (ecstasy) on brain serotonin neurons in human beings." *Lancet* 352(9138) (31 Oct. 1998): 1437.

Moscowitz, N., et al. *Neuropsychopharmacology* 25 (2001): 277–89.

Pfeiffer, C., et al. "Copper, zinc, manganese, niacin and pyridoxine in the schizophrenias." *Journal of Applied Nutrition* 27 (1975): 9–39.

———. "Treatment of pyroluric schizophrenia with large doses of pyridoxine and zinc." *Journal of Orthomolecular Psychiatry* 3 (1974): 292–93.

Reneman, L., et al. "Cortical serotonin transporter density and verbal memory in individuals who stopped using 'ecstasy.'" *Archives of General Psychiatry* 58(10) (2001).

Smith, M., et al. "Psychoactive constituents of the genus sceletium: a review." *Journal of Ethnopharmacology* 50(3) (1996): 119–30.

CHAPTER 9: "ADDICTED?
I CAN QUIT WHENEVER I WANT"

Cummings, S. R., et al. "Epidemiology of osteoporosis and osteoporotic fracture." *Epidemiologic Review* 7 (1985): 178–208.

Cutler, E. *The Food Allergy Cure: A New Solution to Food Cravings, Obesity, Depression, Headaches, Arthritis, and Fatigue.* New York: Harmony Books, 2001.

Drummond, E. *Overcoming Anxiety Without Tranquilizers.* New York: Dutton Books, 1997.

Lader, M. "Benzodiazepines—the opiate of the masses?" *Neuroscience* 3 (1978): 159–65.

———. "Dependence on benzodiazepines." *Journal of Clinical Psychiatry* 44 (1983): 121–27.

Oster, G., et al. "Benzodiazepines and the risk of traffic accidents." *American Journal of Public Health* 80 (1990): 1467–70.

Tinetti, M. E., et al. "Risk factors for falls among elderly persons living in the community." *New England Journal of Medicine* 319 (1988): 1701–7.

References

CHAPTER 11: MOVING TOWARD BLISS

Ichazo, O. *Interviews with Oscar Ichazo*. New York: Arica Institute Press, 1982.
Roth, G. *Sweat Your Prayers: Movement as Spiritual Practice*. New York: Tarcher/ Putnam, 1997.
Silverberg, D. S. "Non-pharmacological treatment of hypertension." *Journal of Hypertension Supplement* 894 (Sept. 1990): 521–26.
Szabo, A., et al. "Phenylethylamine, a possible link to the antidepressant effects of exercise?" *British Journal of Sports Medicine* 35 (2001): 342–43.

CHAPTER 12: THE BREATH OF LIFE AND
CHAPTER 13: MEDITATION AND THE MIND

Delmonte, M. M. "Meditation as a clinical intervention strategy: a brief review." *International Journal of Psychosomatics* (1984): 31.
———. "Physiological concomitants of meditation practice." *International Journal of Psychosomatics* 31 (1984): 23.
Hendricks, G. *Achieving Vibrance*. New York: Harmony Books, 2002.
Keicolt-Glaser, J. K., et al. "Modulation of cellular immunity in medical students." *Journal of Behavioral Medicine* 9 (1986): 5.
Thornton, J. *A Field Guide to the Soul: A Down-to-Earth Handbook of Spiritual Practice*. New York: Bell Tower/Crown Publishers, 1999.

CHAPTER 14: BIOFEEDBACK, RELAXATION,
AND THE ALPHA STATE

Robbins, J. *Symphony in the Brain: The Evolution of the New Brain Wave Biofeedback*. New York: Grove Press, 2001. (Available on www.symphonyinthebrain.com).
Wise, A. *Awakening the Mind: A Guide to Mastering the Power of Your Brain Waves*. New York: Jeremy P. Tarcher, 2002.

CHAPTER 16: THE POWER OF TOUCH

"Neglect Harms Infants' Brains, Researchers Say." *Los Angeles Times*, 28 Oct. 1997.
Oz, M. *Healing from the Heart*. New York: Penguin Books, 1998, p. 106.

References

CHAPTER 17: SEXUAL CHEMISTRY

Cutler, W. "Human sex-attractant pheromones: discovery, research, development and application in sex therapy." *Psychiatric Annals—The Journal of Continuing Psychiatric Education* 20(1) (1999): 54–59.

CHAPTER 20: LIGHT AND COLOR

Downing, D. *Daylight Robbery.* London: Arrow Books, 1988.
Hinkle, L., and H. Wolff. "Ecologic investigation of the relationship between illness, life experiences and the social environment." *Annals of Internal Medicine* 49 (1958): 1373–88.
Lefebure, F. *Phosphenism.* Psychotechnic Publications, 1990.
Pathak, M. "Activation of the melanocyte system by ultraviolet radiation and cell transformation." *Annals of the New York Academy of Sciences* 453 (1985): 328–39.

CHAPTER 21: DEEP SLEEP

Brain/Mind Bulletin (21 Jan. and 11 Feb. 1985) (out of print).
"For Better Learning, Researchers Endorse 'Sleep on It' Adage." *New York Times on the Web* (7 Mar. 2000) (Available on www.nytimes.com/library/national/science/health/030700hth-sleep-memory.html).
Gallup Organization. *Sleep in America: A National Survey of US Adults.* Princeton: National Sleep Foundation, 1998.

Recommended Reading

THE BRAIN

Brain Longevity by Dharma Singh Khalsa, M.D. (Warner Books, 1999).
Change Your Brain, Change Your Life by Daniel Amen, M.D. (Times Books, 1998).
Mind Boosters by Ray Sahelian, M.D. (St. Martin's Press, 2000).
Molecules of Emotion by Candace Pert (Simon & Schuster, 1999).
Smart Drugs and Nutrients, I and II by Ward Dean, M.D., and John Morgenthaler (Smart Publications, 1990, 1993) www.smart-publications.com; Phone: (707) 284-3125.
Why God Won't Go Away: Brain Science and the Biology of Belief by Andrew Newberg, Eugene D'Aquili, and Vince Rause (Ballantine Books, 2002).
Your Miracle Brain by Jean Carper (HarperCollins, 2000).

DIET AND NUTRITION

The ADD Nutrition Solution by Marcia Zimmerman (Henry Holt, 1999).
Caffeine Blues by Stephen Cherniske (Warner Books, 1998).
Crazymakers by Carol Simontacchi (Jeremy P. Tarcher, 2000).
The Diet Cure by Julia Ross (Penguin Putnam, 1999).
Eat Right for Your Type by Peter D'Adamo (Penguin Putnam, 1997).
40-30-30 Diet by Ann Louise Gittleman (Keats Publishing, 1997).
Mastering the Zone by Barry Sears, M.D. (Regan Books, 1997).

Recommended Reading

The Optimum Nutrition Bible by Patrick Holford (Crossing Press, 1998).
Potatoes, Not Prozac by Kathleen Desmaisons (Simon & Schuster, 1998).
The Real Vitamin and Mineral Book, 2d edition, by Shari Lieberman and Nancy Bruning (Avery, 1997).

NATURAL SOLUTIONS FOR STRESS

Kava: Medicine Hunting in Paradise by Chris Kilham (Park Street Press, 1996).
Kava: Nature's Answer to Stress, Anxiety and Insomnia by Hyla Cass, M.D., and Terrence McNally (Prima Publishing, 1998).
Tired of Being Tired by Jesse Hanley, M.D. (Penguin Putnam, 2001).
Waking the Tiger Within by Peter Levine and Ann Frederick (North Atlantic Books, 1997).

NATURAL SOLUTIONS FOR DEPRESSION

End Depression Naturally by Joan Matthews Larson (Random House, 2000).
Prozac Backlash by Joseph Glenmullen, M.D. (Touchstone Books, 2001).
St. John's Wort: Nature's Blues Buster by Hyla Cass, M.D. (Avery, 1997).

PSYCHEDELICS, ENTHEOGENS, AND ALTERED STATES OF CONSCIOUSNESS

DMT—The Spirit Molecule by Rick Strassman, M.D. (Park Street Press, 1999). Also visit www.rickstrassman.com.
The Doors of Perception by Aldous Huxley (Flamingo, 1954).
Ecstasy: The Complete Guide by Julie Holland, M.D. (Park Street Press, 2001).
The Encyclopedia of Psychoactive Substances by Richard Rudgley (Abacus, 1998).
Entheogens and the Future of Religion by Robert Forti (Council on Spiritual Practices, 1997). Also visit www.csp.org.
Lessons from the Light: What We Can Learn from the Near-Death Experience by Evelyn E. Valarino and Kenneth Ring (Monument Point Press, 2000).
Psyche Delicacies by Chris Kilham (Rodale Press, 2001).

MOVEMENT, YOGA

Sweat Your Prayers: Movement as Spiritual Practice by Gabrielle Roth (Tarcher/Putnam, 1997).
Yoga for Dummies by Georg Feuerstein, Larry Payne, and Lilias Folan (IDG Books Worldwide, 1999).

Recommended Reading

INNER WORK

Achieving Vibrance by Gay Hendricks (Harmony Books, 2002).

The Art of Everyday Ecstasy by Margo Anand and Deepak Chopra (Broadway Books, 1998).

In the Footsteps of Gandhi by Catherine Ingram (Parallax Press, 1990).

Inner Peace for Busy People: 52 Simple Strategies for Transforming Your Life by Joan Borysenko, Ph.D. (Hay House, 2001).

MEDITATION

The Best Guide to Meditation by Victor Davich (Renaissance Media, 1998).

Lovingkindness: The Revolutionary Art of Happiness by Sharon Salzberg and Jon Kabat-Zinn (Shambhala Publications, 1997).

Meditation As Medicine by Dharma Singh Khalsa (Pocket Books, 2001). Medical meditation is an adaptation of kundalini yoga combined with meditation, using specific breathing patterns and postures as well as movements, mantras, and mental focus. Audiotape also available.

Meditation Made Easy by Lorin Roche (Harper San Francisco, 1998).

Wherever You Go, There You Are: Mindfulness Meditation in Everyday Life by Jon Kabat-Zinn (Hyperion, 1995).

BIOFEEDBACK, RELAXATION, AND THE ALPHA STATE

Awakening the Mind: A Guide to Mastering the Power of Your Brain Waves by Anna Wise (Tarcher/Putnam, 2002).

The High-Performance Mind: Mastering Brainwaves for Insight, Healing, and Creativity by Anna Wise (Tarcher/Putnam, 1996).

The Relaxation Response by Herbert Benson, M.D. (Wholecare, 2000).

A Symphony in the Brain: The Evolution of the New Brain Wave Biofeedback by Jim Robbins (Atlantic Monthly Press, 2000).

POSITIVE THINKING

Finding Flow by Mihaly Csikszentmihalyi (Basic Books, 1998).

Flow: The Psychology of Optimal Experience by Mihaly Csikszentmihalyi (Harper Collins, 1993).

Getting the Love You Want by Harville Hendrix, Ph.D. (Pocket Books, 1993).

The Seven Spiritual Laws of Success by Deepak Chopra (Amber-Allen, 1995).

What We May Be by Piero Ferrucci (Jeremy P. Tarcher, 1993).

Recommended Reading

You Can Make It Happen: A 9-Step Plan for Success by Graham Stedman (Fireside Books, 1997).

HEALING WITH TOUCH

Healing from the Heart by Mehmet Oz, M.D. (Penguin, 1998).
Massage for Dummies by Steven Capellini and Michel Van Welden (IDG Books Worldwide, 1999).

SEXUAL CHEMISTRY

The Art of Sexual Ecstasy by Margo Anand (Jeremy P. Tarcher, 1998).
Passion Play: Ancient Secrets for a Lifetime of Health and Happiness Through Sensational Sex by Felice Dunas and Philip Goldberg (Riverhead, 1998).
Tantra: The Art of Conscious Loving by Charles and Caroline Muir (Mercury House, 1990).

MUSIC AS THERAPY

The Power of Sound by Joshua Leeds (Healing Arts Press, 2001).
Sounds of Healing: A Physician Reveals the Therapeutic Power of Sound, Voice and Music by Mitchell L. Gaynor, M.D. (Broadway Books, 1999).

ADDICTION

End Your Addiction Now: The Proven Nutritional Supplement Program That Can Set You Free by Charles Gant, M.D. (Warner Books, 2002).
Overcoming Anxiety Without Tranquilizers by Edward Drummond, M.D. (Dutton, 1997).
Prozac Backlash by Joseph Glenmullen, M.D. (Touchstone Books, 2001).
Seven Weeks to Sobriety by Joan Matthews Larson (Fawcett Books, 1997).

INTEGRATIVE MEDICINE, WELLNESS

Healing Myths, Healing Magic: Breaking the Spell of Old Illusions; Reclaiming Our Power to Heal by Donald M. Epstein (Amber-Allen, 2000).

Resources

Resources

American Botanical Council
www.herbalgram.org
Provides up-to-date information on herbal products, including research, uses, and legislative issues.

BLTC Research
www.biopsychiatry.com
Looks at maximizing human potential and promoting well-being through an in-depth understanding of our biochemical programming.

Cognitive Enhancement Research Institute (CERI)
www.ceri.com
A great source for keeping up to date on mind and memory boosters.

Dancesafe
www.dancesafe.org
A nonprofit, harm-reduction organization whose volunteers are trained to be health educators and drug abuse–prevention counselors in their communities.

DORway
www.dorway.com/blayenn.html
Provides scientific information on artificial sweeteners.

Erowid, The Vaults of
www.erowid.org
An online library of information about psychoactive plants and chemicals and related topics, spanning the spectrum from solid peer-reviewed research to fanciful creative writing.

A Healing Touch — Healer Training Schools
with gifted teacher and healer, Ron Lavin, M.A.; www.ahealingtouch.com
Self-healing practices and practitioner training for personal transformational growth and healing of the body, mind, and spirit. (This is a personal recommendation!)

Heffter Research Institute
www.heffter.org
An organization dedicated to researching the effects of entheogens and the frontiers of neuroscience and consciousness.

Hendricks Institute
www.hendricks.com
The Center for Professional Breathwork and Movement offers certification for breath and movement coaches.

INNATE INTELLIGENCE, INC.

www.innateintelligence.com

An innovative thinker and healer, chiropractor Donald Epstein describes his concept of wellness as "the experience of wholeness, invincibility, flexibility, openness to life, and an ability to feel alive." Sure sounds like a natural high!

INTERNATIONAL COALITION FOR DRUG AWARENESS

www.drugawareness.org

800-280-0730

Ann Blake Tracy, Ph.D. in Psychology and Health Sciences, is author of the book Prozac: Panacea or Pandora's Box?, *on adverse reactions to serotonergic medications.*

THE MULTIDISCIPLINARY ASSOCIATION FOR PSYCHEDELIC STUDIES (MAPS)

www.maps.org

A nonprofit research and educational organization that helps scientists to design, fund, obtain approval for, and report on studies into the healing and spiritual potentials of various substances. Its stated goal is "to use the data generated from scientific research to develop these drugs into prescription medicines."

OPTIMAL BREATHING

www.breathing.com

Articles and instruction on Optimal Breathing, an important adjunct to almost any therapy modality.

BIOFEEDBACK, RELAXATION, AND THE ALPHA STATE

ANNA WISE CENTER FOR BRAINWAVE BIOFEEDBACK AND CONSCIOUSNESS DEVELOPMENT

www.annawise.com

1000A Magnolia

Larkspur, CA 94939

415-925-9449

Books, CDs, and training in neurofeedback.

BIOCYBERNAUT INSTITUTE

www.biocybernaut.com

Provides Biocybernaut EEG training.

BRAIN.COM

www.brain.com

Information and products for the brain.

Resources

EEG SPECTRUM INTERNATIONAL, INC.
www.EEGspectrum.com
818-778-6137
News and information on neurofeedback, national list of EEG therapists, and therapist training.

FUTUREHEALTH.ORG
www.futurehealth.org
Information on biofeedback, neurofeedback, and optimal functioning.

SAMADHI TANK COMPANY
www.samadhitank.com
Isolation and flotation tanks.

OPEN FOCUS
www.openfocus.com
Neurofeedback training (and tapes) for optimizing attention; for sports, academics, stress, pain-management training, preventive health care, and biofeedback.

VIBRASOUND TABLE
www.vibrasound.com
The VibraSound® Total Sensory Wave Table is an innovative device for changing your brain frequency.

OTHER MIND-BODY THERAPIES

AROMATHERAPY
www.naturalhealthscience.com
Fax: 360-422-7729
Dr. Bruce Berkowsky, Institute of Natural Health Science
Course, information, and products.

JOSH LEEDS
www.Sound_remedies.com

LIGHT AND COLOR: TOOLS FOR WELLNESS
www.toolsforwellness.com
800-456-9887
Source for alternative health products, including full-spectrum lighting, and other information.

Resources

Q-LINK
www.clarus.com
The Q-Link pendant is based on the emerging science of subtle energies, which has discovered that a pure source of subtle energy can boost human bioenergy. Research also shows that enhanced bioenergy provides extra EMF protection.

STEVEN HALPERN'S INNER PEACE MUSIC
www.innerpeacemusic.com
Information on music as a transformational tool; descriptions and sales of tapes and CDs.

COMPLEMENTARY AND ALTERNATIVE MEDICINE, INCLUDING NATURAL HEALTH PRACTITIONERS

ALTERNATIVE MEDICINE DIGEST
www.AlternativeMedicine.com
An extensive and up-to-date Web site.

THE AMERICAN ASSOCIATION OF NATUROPATHIC PHYSICIANS
www.naturopathic.org
Phone: 877-969-2267

AMERICAN ASSOCIATION OF ORIENTAL MEDICINE
www.aaom.org
Phone: 888-500-7999

AMERICAN HERBALISTS GUILD
AmericanHerbalistsGuild.com
Phone: 770-751-6021

AMERICAN HERBAL PRODUCTS ASSOCIATION (AHPA)
www.ahpa.org
Good source of up-to-date information on herbal safety and use.

AMERICAN HOLISTIC HEALTH ASSOCIATION
www.ahha.org
Maintains a list of practitioner referral sources.

BIOSET®
www.drellencutler.com
Information on BioSet courses and practitioners.

Resources

HEALTH WORLD ONLINE
www.healthy.net
Comprehensive information on complementary and alternative medicine, books, practitioners, and products.

NATURAL TREATMENT FOR ALLERGIES
Nambudripad's Allergy Elimination Technique (NAET)
www.naet.org
Supplies information, list of practitioners, and professional training courses on a natural treatment for allergies.

ORGANIZATIONS FOR SELF-HELP AND FOR INNER TRANSFORMATIONAL WORK

ALCOHOLICS ANONYMOUS
www.alcoholics-anonymous.org
For 12-step programs. Check your local phone book for Alcoholics Anonymous. There are also many other specific 12-step programs, such as Cocaine Anonymous, Overeaters Anonymous, and Gamblers Anonymous.

ARICA INSTITUTE INC.
www.pcals.com
860-927-1006
Provides a contemporary method for the clarification of the human process into states of enlightenment and liberation.

ESALEN INSTITUTE
www.esalen.org
Hwy 1, Big Sur, CA 93920
831-667-3060
One of the original retreat centers for restoration as well as educational and transformational workshops.

HOFFMAN PROCESS, THE HOFFMAN INSTITUTE
www.quadrinity.com
800-506-5253
A week-long residential course that deals with negative patterns of behavior that we inherit from childhood. The course leads to transformation in relating and relationships.

Resources

INSTITUTE OF HEARTMATH®
www.heartmath.com

HeartMath has shown how decision making from the heart can modulate and entrain our overactive and often misperceiving brains, with the results being more holistic and, ultimately, more effective. Leading with the heart may be the right way to go after all!

LANDMARK EDUCATION
The Landmark Forum
www.landmarkeducation.com

A three-day course providing rapid, profound transformation for living life fully and effectively in those areas of life that are important to you. Centers all over the world, including in most major U.S. cities.

LIFE PATH RETREATS
www.Lifepathretreats.com
888-667-3873

Journeys of self-discovery, held in picturesque San Miguel de Allende, Mexico.

OMEGA INSTITUTE FOR HOLISTIC STUDIES
www.eomega.org
150 Lake Drive
Rhinebeck, NY 12572
845-266-4444
Fax: 845-266-3769

Pioneering growth center in the beautiful Catskill Mountains provides workshops and retreats. Also holds conferences in various other locations.

PSYCHOCALISTHENICS
www.pcals.com
415-383-6097

Books, audio- and videotapes, and classes. You can teach yourself by ordering the self-tuition kit: the book Master Level Exercise: Psychocalisthenics *by Oscar Ichazo, a video, a wall, chart, and a music cassette with voice guide.*

TAICHI
www.thetaichisite.com *and* www.taichifoundation.org
For news, classes, books, and videos worldwide.

Resources

WHITE LOTUS FOUNDATION
www.whitelotus.org
2500 San Marco Pass
Santa Barbara, CA 93105
805-964-1944
Ganga White and Tracy Rich, renowned founders of this yoga teacher training and retreat center, have also created excellent instruction videotapes, including their famous Double Yoga—do it with a friend!

YOGA ALLIANCE
www.yogaalliance.org
877-964-2255
Yoga Alliance provides support services for yoga professionals and maintains a national registry of teachers.

MEDITATION RETREATS AND INSTRUCTION

Buddhist Meditation

INSIGHT MEDITATION SOCIETY
www.dharma.org
978-355-4378
Long- and short-term retreats; workshops, classes, books, and tapes by Buddhist teacher and author Sharon Salzberg.

SPIRIT ROCK
www.spiritrock.org
415-488-0164
Long- and short-term retreats; workshops, classes, books, and tapes.

TRICYCLE.COM
Listings of retreat centers, books, and tapes, and a newsletter.

Resources

Other Types of Meditation

DHARMA DIALOGUES WITH CATHERINE INGRAM
www.dharmadialogues.org
Instructional talks, retreats, and tapes.

SIDDHA YOGA CENTERS
www.siddhayoga.org
Courses and further information on this form of meditation, first introduced to the West by Swami Muktananda.

Spas

No longer just a luxury for the rich, spas of all types are rapidly increasing in popularity as resources for healing the mind, body, and spirit. In addition to some rare peace and quiet, resort and destination spas offer an amazing array of healing treatments and transformational activities that go far beyond what you might expect. Additionally, there are increasing numbers of day spas that many people use for a weekly renewal or just an occasional time away from it all. If you haven't tried one before, you might be surprised at the benefits from just a bit of time-out. Most of us living in this increasingly stressed-out world not only deserve it, we need it! Check your local listings, or get recommendations from friends.

CANYON RANCH
www.canyonranch.com
A world-class spa that attends to the mind, body, and spirit of its guests.

HEALING RETREATS AND SPAS
www.healingretreats.com
A monthly magazine that, besides providing informative articles, keeps you apprised of available spa retreats and activities.

ROYAL TREATMENT
www.royaltreatment.com
Steve Capellini (author of Massage for Dummies *and* The Royal Treatment*) provides a good resource for spa information on his Web site.*

Resources

SUPPLEMENT SUPPLIERS

ALLERGY RESEARCH GROUP/NUTRICOLOGY
www.nutricology.com
800-405-4274
Full catalog of high-quality, hypo-allergenic supplements.

BODHI TREE BOOKSTORE
www.bodhitree.com
Another all-time favorite of mine, for books and New Age accessories as well as enlightening lectures by popular authors.

ELIXIR TONICS & TEAS
www.elixir.net
8612 Melrose Ave.
Los Angeles, CA 90069
310-657-9300
Provides high-quality herbal products in a unique and beautiful setting. It is also across the street from the famous Bodhi Tree Bookstore.

INTERNATIONAL ACADEMY OF COMPOUNDING PHARMACISTS
www.healthy.net/professionals/compound.asp
800-927-4227
Lists compounding pharmacists who supply prescription items such as L-tryptophan and natural hormones that are not generally carried by regular pharmacies.

NATURAL BALANCE
www.naturalbalance.com
Manufactures supplements that promote good mood and high energy. Our favorite is the Happy Camper kava blend.

NORTH AMERICAN HERB AND SPICE COMPANY
www.biobalance.tv
800-243-5242
Provides a variety of high-quality herbals, including an outstanding St. John's wort product.

Resources

Index

Index

Index

Index

Light, 273–274
  colors, 274–275
Lilly, John, Dr., 238
Limbic system, 258
Lobstein, Dennis, Dr., 218
L-phenylalanine, 103
LSD, 165, 168–170
L-tryptophan, 124–125, 281

Magic mushrooms. *See* Psilocybin mushrooms
Mantra, 234
Marijuana, 59–62
Massage, 249–253
Mastering the Zone (Sears), 40
Maté, 87–88
Mayans, 164–165
McCraty, Rollin, Dr., 245
Measures, 7
Meditation, 233–235
  integrating brain with, 235–237
Melatonin, 21, 23, 279–280
Memory boosters. *See* Mind and memory
    boosters
Memory Check (questionnaire), 16–17, 136
Meridians, 223
Mesembrine, 185
Milk thistle, 204
Mind and memory boosters, 136
  action plan for, 159–160
  age-related cognitive decline, 137–138
  declining mental function, 136
  natural mind and memory boosters, 141–
    158
  reversing memory loss, 139–140
  smart drugs and hormones, 140
  stress-related memory loss, 138–139
  synergy from combining, 158–159
Mind-body connection, 4–6
Mind Mirror, 240–241
Minerals, 43, 132, 180
Monoamine oxidase inhibitors (MAOIs),
    119
Mood Check (questionnaire), 15–16, 112
Mood enhancers, 111
  action plan for, 133–135
  antidepressants, 117–120
  aromatherapy as, 261
  and endorphins, 218–219
  mood check, 112
  natural, 120–133
  nutrients for brain, 112–116
Movement, 217
  dancing, 222
  exercise and endorphin release, 218–219
  inner, 222–223
  psychocalisthenics, 221

t'ai chi, 220–221
vital energy enhancers, 224–225
yoga, 219–220
Multivitamin/mineral formula, high-potency,
    44–45
Music, 267
  chemistry of sound, 269–270
  ecstasy through, 270–271
  rhythm entrainment, 268–269
  selections chart, 271–272
Myelin sheath, 40

NADH, 108, 297
NAET (Nambudripad's Allergy Elimination
    Technique), 197
Natural highs
  basics for, 29–45, 211–216
  connectors for, 173–187
  energizers for, 94–110
  four steps to, 11–12
  mind and memory boosters, 141–158
  mood enhancers, 120–133
  questionnaires, 12–18
  sleep aids, 279–281
  A to Z list of, 290–303
Net protein usability (NPU), 36
Neurofeedback, 238–241
Neurons, 19
Neurotransmitters, 5–6, 19–24, 31, 114–116,
    145, 162, 198
New England Journal of Medicine, 43, 90
Nicotine, 201
Nootropics, 140
Noradrenaline, 21–22, 115–116
Nucleus accumbens, 22
Nutrition. *See also* Antioxidants; Minerals;
    Vitamins; Water
  amino acids, 23–25
  balance in, 40–41
  for brain, 11
  and brain chemistry, 11, 23–25, 112–116,
    141–158
  carbohydrates, 30–31, 40
  essential fatty acids, 27–28, 38–39
  as fuel, 29–30
  protein, 31, 36–38

O'Callahan, James, 172
Omega-3 fats, 39, 41, 131, 148–150
Omega-6 fats, 39, 151
Optimum Nutrition Bible (Holford), 41
Osmond, Humphrey, 178
Oxygen, 42
Oxygenation of body, 227–228
Oxytocin, 255
Oz, Mehmet, Dr., 249

Index